23

W9-AUZ-294

# 100 Questions & Answers About Gastroesophageal Reflux Disease (GERD): *A Lahey Clinic Guide*

David L. Burns, MD, CNSP
*Department of Gastroenterology*
*Lahey Clinic*
*Burlington, MA*

Neeral L. Shah, MD
*Department of Gastroenterology*
*Lahey Clinic*
*Burlington, MA*

JONES AND BARTLETT PUBLISHERS
*Sudbury, Massachusetts*
BOSTON    TORONTO    LONDON    SINGAPORE

*World Headquarters*
Jones and Bartlett Publishers
40 Tall Pine Drive
Sudbury, MA 01776
978-443-5000
info@jbpub.com
www.jbpub.com

Jones and Bartlett Publishers
Canada
6339 Ormindale Way
Mississauga, Ontario
L5V 1J2
CANADA

Jones and Bartlett Publishers
International
Barb House, Barb Mews
London W6 7PA
UK

Jones and Bartlett's books and products are available through most bookstores and online booksellers. To contact Jones and Bartlett Publishers directly, call 800-832-0034, fax 978-443-8000, or visit our website at www.jbpub.com.

Substantial discounts on bulk quantities of Jones and Bartlett's publications are available to corporations, professional associations, and other qualified organizations. For details and specific discount information, contact the special sales department at Jones and Bartlett via the above contact information or send an email to specialsales@jbpub.com.

The authors, editor, and publisher have made every effort to provide accurate information. However, they are not responsible for errors, omissions, or for any outcomes related to the use of the contents of this book and take no responsibility for the use of the products and procedures described. Treatments and side effects described in this book may not be applicable to all people; likewise, some people may require a dose or experience a side effect that is not described herein. Drugs and medical devices are discussed that may have limited availability controlled by the Food and Drug Administration (FDA) for use only in a research study or clinical trial. Research, clinical practice, and government regulations often change the accepted standard in this field. When consideration is being given to use of any drug in the clinical setting, the health care provider or reader is responsible for determining FDA status of the drug, reading the package insert, and reviewing prescribing information for the most up-to-date recommendations on dose, precautions, and contraindications, and determining the appropriate usage for the product. This is especially important in the case of drugs that are new or seldom used.

**Library of Congress Cataloging-in-Publication Data**
Burns, David L.
100 questions & answers about gastroesophageal reflux disease (GERD): a Lahey Clinic guide / David L. Burns, Neeral L. Shah.
p. cm.
Includes bibliographical references and index.
ISBN-13: 978-0-7637-4047-4 (alk. paper)
ISBN-10: 0-7637-4047-0 (alk. paper)
1. Gastroesophageal reflux—Miscellanea. 2. Gastroesophageal reflux
—Popular works. I. Shah, Neeral L. II. Lahey Clinic. III. Title.
IV. Title: One hundred questions & answers about gastroesophageal reflux disease (GERD). V. Title: 100 questions and answers about gastroesophageal reflux disease (GERD).
RC815.7.B87 2007
616.3'24—dc22

2006016491

6048

**Production Credits**
Executive Editor: Christopher Davis
Production Director: Amy Rose
Associate Production Editor: Rachel Rossi
Associate Editor: Kathy Richardson
Associate Marketing Manager: Laura Kavigian
Manufacturing Buyer: Amy Bacus
Composition: Northeast Compositors, Inc.
Cover Design: Kate Ternullo
Printing and Binding: Malloy, Inc.
Cover Printing: Malloy, Inc.

Printed in the United States of America
10 09 08 07 06   10 9 8 7 6 5 4 3 2 1

# Contents

**Contents**

# Acknowledgments

This book would not have been possible without the support of Jones and Bartlett Publishers and Executive Publisher Christopher Davis. I am also appreciative of the contribution of one of my patients, Mr. Richard Auth, whose unique understanding of GERD has been inspiring.

I am thankful for the support, love, and patience of my family, my wife Margo Moskos, MD, and our children, Stacy and Alex, in the preparation of this book. I am also thankful to my parents, Hedy and Arthur Burns, who were there for me through it all. They have had chronic heartburn forever, which I may have contributed to.

David L. Burns, MD

I would like to thank my parents, Lalit and Surekha, my family, and my friends for all of their support through the many years of medical education and training. Without their support, I would not have accomplished all that I have, neither would I have had the opportunity to write this book. To all of you, with the utmost sincerity, thank you.

Neeral L. Shah, MD

Gastroesophageal reflux disease or heartburn affects all of us at sometime. About one-third of Americans experience reflux symptoms with some regularity. For a gastroenterologist, reflux and its complications are two of the most common problems managed in the clinic, and the most common reason patients are referred for upper endoscopy. There are many myths regarding the causes and treatment of heartburn. The purpose of this book is to dispel some of the myths and explain the facts. Many feel that reflux is a benign problem and an annoyance. This may be true for some; however, it is a very common reason for doctor's appointments and consumes many millions of dollars in over-the-counter and prescription drugs. Further, reflux truly is not a benign process; it has complications that include temporary or permanent acid damage to the esophagus. Certain cancers of the esophagus are associated with chronic heartburn. And as doctors, we are starting to understand the contribution of GERD symptoms to chronic cough and asthma.

Thankfully, there are some easy ways to improve heartburn symptoms. These may be changes in one's lifestyle or can involve medications. These are all discussed in this book, including the different kinds of medications, their route of action, appropriate usage, and when to take the medication. There are also many issues and misconceptions about the medical and surgical procedures that are done in an attempt to improve reflux symptoms. Recently, new nonsurgical procedures have become available for GERD; we wanted to review and discuss each of these individually; focusing on long-term benefits like eliminating or reducing the need for medications and complications associated with each procedure.

We wrote this book for several reasons. We deal with GERD and its complications daily in medical practice and wanted to have a guide covering the entire spectrum of disease and all of its treatment options including appropriate diagnosis, treatment, and what to do if all fails. On a personal level, I (DLB) have had daily heartburn symptoms for over 20 years and can empathize with my patients and explain how I have dealt with symptoms.

Our hope is that this book is educational and explains some of the issues dealing with chronic GERD including: causes, complications, evaluation, medications, and surgical and medical treatment. It was written to explain the issues on a patient level rather than in "med speak." We certainly learned a lot while preparing this book and will incorporate our improved understanding to the practice of medicine.

*David L. Burns, MD*
*Neeral L. Shah, MD*

# PART ONE

# Gastroesophageal Reflux Disease: Definitions and Facts

What is gastroesophageal reflux disease, or GERD?

Is GERD serious?

What are some of the typical symptoms of GERD?

*More...*

# 1. What is gastroesophageal reflux disease, or GERD?

*GERD* is an abbreviation for gastroesophageal reflux disease. **GERD** has several manifestations. Classically, it can be a sensation of warmth or burning in the chest, which can be a mild discomfort to frank pain. You might regurgitate bitter material or burp it up into your mouth. These symptoms are caused by acidic stomach material refluxing from the stomach into the **esophagus**, which is the food pipe (Figure 1).

**Reflux** can occur during the day or at night while you're asleep. Several factors prevent reflux, among them is gravity and the fact that when you are upright,

> *GERD is an abbreviation for gastro-esophageal reflux disease.*

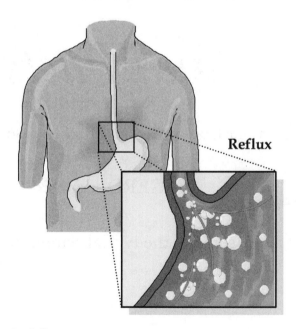

**Figure 1    Reflux.**

the esophagus is above the stomach. GERD symptoms increase particularly at bedtime because the effects and benefits of gravity are removed when you lie down. Generally, nocturnal or nighttime symptoms are more severe; in addition to burning chest discomfort, they can include excessive drooling, coughing, and choking. These symptoms can increase the risks of complications of chronic GERD that may affect the esophagus, lungs, or airways.

Reflux is affected by weight, diet, medications, and lifestyle habits such as smoking and alcohol consumption. A patient with GERD can change or modify many of these factors to improve symptoms. If conservative measures fail, then many medications are available for treatment of GERD. The spectrum of medications spans from over-the-counter **antacids** used to treat infrequent and episodic reflux, to powerful prescription drugs that you take several times a day to treat severe GERD and its complications.

*Reflux is affected by weight, diet, medications, and lifestyle habits such as smoking and alcohol consumption.*

Patients and doctors may use several names for gastroesophageal reflux disease interchangeably. **Heartburn**, acid reflux, and **regurgitation** are all symptoms of GERD. These symptoms are discussed further throughout this book and can be referenced in specific questions.

Richard's comment:

*My acid reflux symptoms are most severe while sleeping. I wake up from a sound sleep with the sensation that I am drowning. The bitter taste stays with me for the rest of the night.*

## 2. What is heartburn?

Heartburn is discomfort or pain in the chest that is caused by acid in the esophagus. It is a manifestation of how pain is felt in the esophagus. Heartburn feels like burning, warmth, or pain in the midchest area. Although heartburn, a symptom of reflux, often feels like burning and can be very similar to the pain or discomfort caused by heart problems or heart attacks, heartburn does not affect the heart, as its name suggests. The reason is that the esophagus passes through the chest almost directly behind the heart, so pain in this area can easily be confused with pain caused by heart problems (see Figures 2 and 2a). Occasionally, the pain is so similar that people actually need to undergo testing to prove the pain is caused by acid in the esophagus and not by a heart attack.

*Although heartburn, a symptom of reflux, often feels like burning and can be very similar to the pain or discomfort caused by heart problems or heart attacks, heartburn does not affect the heart, as its name suggests.*

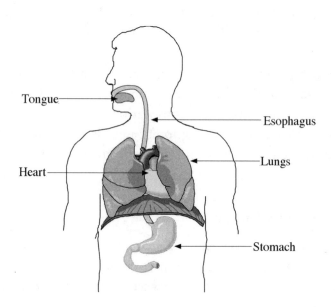

**Figure 2    Digestive System.**

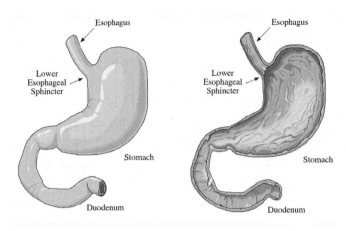

**Figure 2a    Anatomy of a normal esophagus, stomach, and duodenum. (Cut away view on right)**

## 3. What is acid reflux?

Acid for digestion of food is normally produced in the stomach in response to eating. Normally, acid can reflux, or move up, into the esophagus, but protective mechanisms are in place to remove or neutralize refluxed acid. These include saliva, which neutralizes acid, and esophageal pumping, which moves refluxed acid back down to the stomach. Acid reflux disease occurs when increased or prolonged episodes of reflux overwhelm the protective factors, resulting in symptoms.

Excessive acid sitting in the esophagus causes burning discomfort and, in about half of those with chronic symptoms, damage to the esophagus. A bitter or acidic taste can be a manifestation of high reflux called regurgitation. Regurgitation can cause mouth, dental, sinus, and lung problems.

Gastroesophageal reflux disease (GERD) is a disease that is caused by a combination of symptoms. These symptoms can include heartburn, regurgitation,

*Gastroesopha-
geal reflux
disease
(GERD) is a
disease that is
caused by a
combination
of symptoms.
These
symptoms can
include heart-
burn,
regurgitation,
chest pain or
discomfort,
bitter taste in
the mouth,
and difficulty
swallowing.*

chest pain or discomfort, bitter taste in the mouth, and difficulty swallowing. Chronic GERD results from repeated reflux generally defined as symptoms occurring in three or more episodes a week for 6 months or longer. Chronic GERD is associated with damage to the esophagus, which can manifest as inflammation called **esophagitis** and as **ulcers**, and it can predispose a patient to esophageal cancer. Thus, patients with chronic GERD should undergo a prompt evaluation by a doctor to ensure that no complications or damage has occurred.

## 4. How many people are affected by GERD?

GERD is not a new disease; it is a common disease that affects many people. In 1994, the U.S. Department of Health and Human Services reported that about 7 million people in the United States at that time suffered from chronic GERD. That number has grown since, likely because of the increasing incidence of obesity and people being overweight, which are contributing factors to reflux problems. These days, Americans work longer hours, buy more fast food, and eat on the run. Poor dietary habits and the easy availability of fast food at any hour of the day have to increased GERD. Unfortunately, these factors have also caused more obesity, diabetes, heart disease, cholesterol problems, high blood pressure, and strokes, as well.

*Approximately
one in three
Americans
experiences
occasional
GERD as
called by any
of these names.*

Gastroesophageal reflux goes by several names that are used interchangeably, such as GERD, reflux, heartburn, and indigestion. Approximately one in three Americans experiences occasional GERD as called by any of these names.

GERD does not affect any specific demographic group across the United States. In 2003, a national survey by the National Heartburn Alliance showed how common the symptom of heartburn was across the United States. The following ranking of cities and variability of GERD is likely related to the risk of obesity in these cities, which roughly parallels the incidence of GERD. The data were taken from *http://www.-heartburnalliance.org/nosection/top24CityResults.jsp.*

## America's Top 24 Heartburn Cities in 2003

1. Charlotte, NC
2. Jacksonville, FL
3. Roanoke, VA
4. Louisville, KY
5. Denver, CO
6. Spokane, WA
7. Miami, FL
8. Tampa-St. Petersburg, FL
9. Atlanta, GA
10. Grand Rapids, MI
11. Orlando, FL
12. Minneapolis-St. Paul, MN
13. Milwaukee, WI
14. Pittsburgh, PA
15. Boston, MA
16. Raleigh, NC
17. Baltimore, MD
18. Albany, NY
19. Salt Lake City, UT
20. Columbus, OH

21. Cincinnati, OH
22. Omaha, NE
23. Des Moines, IA
24. Peoria, IL

Surveys conducted by national organizations such as the American College of Gastroenterology (ACG) report that the majority of Americans suffer from heartburn or GERD, and symptoms can affect quality of life, sense of health, and enjoyment of food. Eating large or spicy meals often can lead to acid reflux. When heartburn occurs regularly, people may lose their taste for certain foods or become afraid to try new foods for fear of developing symptoms again.

The ACG survey states that more than half of all Americans experience some nighttime reflux symptoms that affect sleep and that prevent many from getting a full night's rest. Experiencing poor-quality sleep or delayed sleep can cause people to feel daytime fatigue and can affect overall health and work or school functioning or productivity.

---

*GERD is affected by many different factors. It can be caused by factors out of your control as well as other factors that you can change or eliminate.*

---

Richard's comment:

*I have found that whenever I discuss my acid reflux condition in a group I am amazed at the number of people have similar symptoms. It would appear to me that there is a tremendous number of sufferers out there.*

## 5. What factors cause GERD?

GERD is affected by many different factors. It can be caused by factors out of your control as well as other factors that you can change or eliminate. A major cause of

GERD and regurgitation is an incompetent valve, or barrier, between the esophagus and stomach. The circular muscle at the bottom of the esophagus is called the **lower esophageal sphincter (LES)**. The LES contributes to the high-pressure zone at the junction of the esophagus and stomach that keeps ingested material out of the esophagus once it has passed through the sphincter. Other components of the high-pressure zone include the ligaments that hold the stomach in place and the **diaphragm**, which is the muscle separating the chest and abdomen. A **hiatal hernia (or hiatus hernia)** is a defect in this zone, when the ligaments are loosened and the top of the stomach moves inappropriately into the chest area (see Figure 3). The development of a hiatal hernia decreases the strength of the LES and promotes reflux.

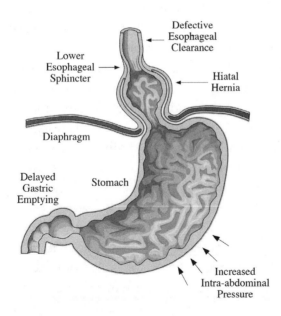

**Figure 3    Hiatal Hernia.**

Hiatal hernias likely are the greatest contributor to or cause of GERD.

Factors out of a patient's control include genetics and personal background. Some people have a family history of GERD that is passed on through genes. People may have family members across several generations who are affected by GERD because of a genetic component. Other inherited factors are body weight and tendency toward obesity. These characteristics tend to run in families and are further contributions to the development of reflux. Sometimes, however, genetic predisposition to a disease can be confused with other family factors. For instance, GERD in family members may be caused by family members who eat the same types of foods or develop the same eating or exercise habits, and not necessarily by a genetic factor.

Other factors called lifestyle choices are within your control; you can change your choices to decrease your symptoms of GERD. Keep in mind that some lifestyle modifications are easier said than done because they are habits that you have developed over years. You might find it necessary to modify these lifestyle issues slowly over time. Lifestyle factors include such choices as limiting alcohol, losing weight, quitting smoking, avoiding certain medications, limiting carbonated beverages, eating smaller meals, and being careful about eating habits (i.e., avoiding spicy, fatty, and fried foods, etc.). Caffeine consumption increases GERD because it relaxes the LES that protects the esophagus from backflow of acidic stomach contents. Caffeine is one lifestyle factor that can easily be reduced, and caffeine is not just contained in coffee; most teas, hot or iced, and many sodas contain caffeine, so it is important for you to read the label to identify foods and drinks that may make your GERD symptoms worse.

New cases of GERD are commonly associated with recent weight gain. In the United States, the epidemic of obesity is likely related to easy availability of food, low cost of food, and the opportunity to "super size" your meals. Obesity causes secondary problems, including complicating diseases such as diabetes, high blood pressure, stroke, heart disease, cancer, elevated cholesterol, and GERD.

*New cases of GERD are commonly associated with recent weight gain.*

Because food is readily available, people may eat one large meal a day rather than three smaller meals. A full or overstuffed stomach is subject to increased pressure and takes longer to empty. Foods high in fat content also slow stomach emptying, giving more opportunity for contents to backflow into the esophagus. The eating habits of Americans are changing. Increasingly, people eat meals at irregular hours rather than at relatively fixed times each day. Normally, we might eat our last meal of the day, and then remain upright for several hours so that gravity helps keep fluid and food down in the stomach. Eating within 2 hours of bedtime increases reflux by adding "more fuel to the fire" by providing material to reflux as well as a stimulus for acid production. Thus, the lack of gravity works against you at night when you lie flat in bed.

The reasons given here are only a small number of all the factors that explain why people suffer from GERD.

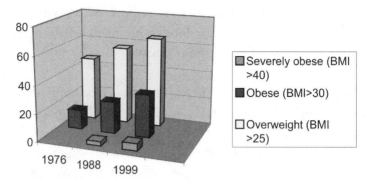

**Figure 4    Obesity in the United States.**

# 6. Is there a link between obesity and GERD in the United States?

*Two-thirds of Americans are overweight, and 1 in 3 are obese or about 30 pounds overweight and at increased risk of obesity-related disease.*

The average body weight of Americans is slowly going up. Obesity is becoming a major issue in our society, starting in young children and continuing through adulthood (See Figure 4.). Two-thirds of Americans are overweight, and 1 in 3 are obese or about 30 pounds overweight and at increased risk of obesity-related disease. The number of obese and morbid obese (100 pounds over your normal weight) people is increasing annually and is considered an epidemic. Changes in the American diet are responsible. Food is cheap and available. Portion size is increasing in an attempt to give the consumer better value and to attract more customers. Food is more calorie dense, meaning it contains more calories per portion and includes more fat and sugar. Sugar-laden sodas are ubiquitous and are marketed directly to children, creating a generation of people addicted to "liquid candy."

The world moves at a faster pace and people are affected by time constraints and convenience. Work and home commitments cause people to make certain sacrifices, such as forgoing the time it takes to prepare wholesome meals and eat at regular intervals. People have less time to eat and exercise; they drive to work and use elevators, which decreases the amount of activity they do. Eating is a major part of our lifestyle, but with less time available in busy days, people are less likely to prepare their own food. Fast food and eating out in restaurants are becoming mainstays of our everyday lives. Prepared foods tend to have higher fat content and contain more preservatives, which can require more stomach acid for proper digestion. This combined with decreased activity levels can lead to weight issues and simply worsen the obesity epidemic in the United States.

Extra body weight within the abdomen puts more pressure on the stomach forcing material back up into the esophagus. Increased food consumption requires more processing and digestion by the gut, compounding the problem and leading to heartburn symptoms. The increasing average weight combined with lifestyle choices has not only led to an obesity epidemic, but also contributes to the increasing problem of **GERD** in the United States.

Richard's comment:

*It has become apparent to me that as my weight increases and my exercise regime decreases, my incidents of nighttime acid reflux go up dramatically. I can only assume that the weight and lack of activity put additional stress on the lower esophageal sphincter (LES). The added weight makes my clothes tightfitting, especially around my stomach, and just adds to my overall physical discomfort.*

## 7. Do children get GERD?

*Yes, children can also get GERD; it can affect anyone.*

Yes, children can also get GERD; it can affect anyone. Infants may exhibit symptoms different from adults. They may become irritable after eating, repeatedly belch or vomit, or suffer from persistent coughing. These symptoms may manifest as poor feeding and impaired weight gain or colic. GERD is often overlooked in young children because their symptoms are very subtle and infants often outgrow the condition.

Parents can take precautions to prevent GERD symptoms in infants, such as keeping infants upright for 30 minutes after feeding instead of placing them directly in the crib. Also, burping the baby more frequently during feeding time can help to avoid the buildup of gas and pressure that may add to a baby's GERD discomfort. If you feed your baby formula, consider changing the formula to reduce symptoms; you should discuss this decision with your child's doctor. If these simple measures do not help, medications may be in order. Some **H2 blockers** and **proton pump inhibitors (PPIs)** are approved by the Food and Drug Administration (FDA) for use in children.

Children experiencing reflux can exhibit typical symptoms, such as heartburn and regurgitation, or atypical symptoms. Frequently, children with asthma have GERD that may be silent and they exhibit no GERD symptoms. These children can require multiple medications for asthma. A trial of antacid medication can be helpful in improving asthma symptoms or decrease the need for asthma medications. You can discuss this with your pediatrician.

As children become older, they can make lifestyle modifications similar to the ones mentioned for adults (i.e., avoiding carbonated beverages, avoiding alcohol, eating dinner early, etc.) to reduce their GERD symptoms.

Richard's comment:

*Because of my history with GERD, I have become very cognizant of how and when my four grandchildren have their meals and what they are eating. While they are small children, I try to get their parents and others to limit unhealthy foods and food habits and emphasize the need for good nutrition. It is so very important to instill healthy habits early in childhood.*

## 8. Does GERD affect one gender more than the other?

Females are slightly more affected by GERD than males are. The reason women are more prone to develop GERD may be related to female hormones. The female body produces the hormones estrogen and progesterone. One of the many functions of these hormones is to relax muscles in the body. For example, during pregnancy, women produce larger amounts of these hormones to relax the muscles in the uterus to allow it to grow along with the baby. Just as hormone levels change during pregnancy, women experience hormonal variations on a regular basis.

*Females are slightly more affected by GERD than males are. The reason women are more prone to develop GERD may be related to female hormones.*

Hormones circulate throughout the body in the blood. When parts of the body are exposed to the hormones, including the muscles in the gastrointestinal tract, they are affected. Under the influence of estrogen and progesterone, the esophagus and stomach relax slightly, affecting their ability to do their job. The esophagus takes the food from the mouth and delivers it to the stomach for further digestion. As the esophagus relaxes, the food moves more slowly down to the stomach, thus increasing the time during which the esophagus can be affected by acid reflux. Similarly, the stomach muscles relax and food stays in the stomach a longer period of time, thus increasing the amount of acid released and the amount of time in which it can reflux. Finally, the lower esophageal sphincter relaxes, allowing esophageal reflux to occur.

Because of all these reasons, women suffer from GERD slightly more than men do.

## 9. Is GERD serious?

*GERD is a serious disease when it goes untreated or is ignored.*

GERD is a serious disease when it goes untreated or is ignored. It can cause occasional or daily problems that are noticeable as a result of pain or discomfort. Reflux disease can be silent or can manifest with atypical symptoms.

Frequent episodes often cause pain or suffering in a patient's everyday life. Untreated chronic GERD can lead to damage of the esophagus. Typical esophageal complications may be inflammation of the esophageal lining, narrowing of the esophagus that leads to difficulty swallowing, or inflammatory conditions predisposing a person to esophageal cancer. Complications of reflux can involve other organ systems, including the sinuses, ears, airways, and lungs.

The risks and specific complications of gastroesophageal reflux disease are extensive, and Part Five, Complications of Gastrointestinal Reflux Disease, in this book discusses these issues.

## 10. What are some of the typical symptoms of GERD?

The major symptoms of GERD include heartburn, chest pain, sour taste in your mouth, and painful or difficult swallowing.

The major or typical symptom of GERD is heartburn, but this can vary among individuals. GERD symptoms fall on a spectrum: for some they are mild or silent, and for others they can be severe. Heartburn is the feeling described as stomach contents and acid travel up into the chest area. The mildest symptoms may be just a slight sense of uneasiness and burning in the chest that occurs only after meals. You might experience a sour taste in your mouth or have bad breath caused by repeated small amounts of acid coming back up into the mouth. A burning sensation behind the breastbone in the chest can be accompanied by a feeling of nausea or uneasiness. Some people experience a burning or a gnawing discomfort in the pit of their stomachs. In severe cases, GERD can cause pain that may be mistaken for a heart attack.

One symptom patients find very disturbing is regurgitation of stomach contents and acid. This can manifest as burping with a bitter taste in the mouth. The most severe type of regurgitation is when you wake at night choking after you have regurgitated a large amount of fluid and inhaled it into your lungs. This can result in shortness of breath, choking, coughing, worsening chronic lung disease, or even pneumonia, which can be life-threatening.

Painful or difficult swallowing is not uncommon and warrants a doctor's evaluation. Repeated regurgitation

*The major symptoms of GERD include heartburn, chest pain, sour taste in your mouth, and painful or difficult swallowing.*

of acid contents can inflame the lining of the esophagus and cause ulcers or other irritation. Swallowed food passes through irritated areas and can cause pain. When the irritated areas heal, these damaged cells are replaced but scarring may result in narrowing of the esophagus, a condition called a **stricture** or **lower esophageal ring**. This narrowing of the esophagus can cause difficulty swallowing, and you might experience it as the sensation of food becoming stuck in your throat or chest.

## 11. What causes new-onset GERD?

*Many different factors can contribute to the development and presence of acid reflux.*

GERD is a disease that is caused by stomach acid abnormally moving up into the esophagus and possibly higher into the mouth or airway structures. Many different factors can contribute to the development and presence of acid reflux.

Normally, your body's natural protective factors limit reflux. We produce 1 pint to 1 quart of saliva per day that is swallowed. Saliva has many jobs. Saliva neutralizes acid, which means it buffers any acid that refluxes into the esophagus. It also helps to digest food, protect the teeth, and lubricate the esophagus so we can swallow. We swallow hundreds of times a day. The purpose of a swallow is to move material from the mouth to the esophagus and ultimately to the stomach. Frequently, swallowing occurs spontaneously without our intentional control. This spontaneous swallowing is protective against reflux because it clears material from the esophagus, including refluxed acid that may be present. Decreased saliva production either as a consequence of aging or because you are taking medications can be a contributing factor to new-onset GERD.

Also, if your esophageal muscle is weak, it may decrease clearance of refluxed acid from the esophagus.

Gravity passively protects the esophagus from material moving up from the stomach, but there are local factors. Normally, there is an anatomic barrier to reflux. This barrier is made up of several structures that are at the junction of the stomach and esophagus. But first, a short anatomy lesson. The **diaphragm** is a muscle that separates the chest from the abdomen and enables us to breathe. The esophagus passes from the chest into the abdomen through a hole, or **hiatus**. Fibrous tissues in the abdomen called ligaments hold the stomach and esophagus in place. At the bottom of the esophagus within its wall is a circular band of muscle called the **lower esophageal sphincter (LES)**. This muscle is usually contracted or closed between swallows to prevent movement of material down to the stomach or up from the stomach, as in reflux. When you swallow, this muscle relaxes and allows food material to pass from the esophagus to the stomach. The LES blocks reflux by staying closed.

This normal anatomy is required to maintain normal esophageal function because the diaphragm, ligaments, and circular muscle all contribute to the amount of pressure the LES can generate to block reflux. Normal anatomy can be lost as part of the aging process. The ligaments can stretch and the hole, or hiatus, in the diaphragm can enlarge. If this happens, part of the stomach can move up into the chest instead of normally staying in the abdomen. This condition is called a hiatus or hiatal hernia (see Figure 5). Because the normal relationships between the structures that contribute to the strength of the lower esophageal sphinc-

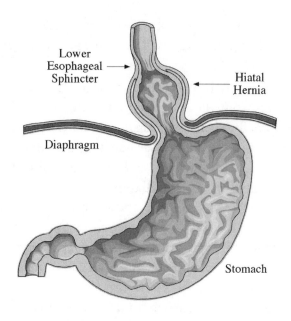

**Figure 5    Hiatal Hernia Only.**

ter are lost, the LES loses its ability to remain contracted with its normal strength, and the result is reflux.

Weight gain and obesity increase the risk of developing acid reflux disease. Extra body weight within the wall of the abdomen leaves less room within the abdominal cavity and increases pressure on the stomach. Increased pressure within the abdomen counteracts the benefits of gravity as a protective factor against reflux. Similarly, a pregnant woman's enlarged uterus, which takes up space in the abdomen, can also push the stomach and its contents up into the esophagus, causing reflux. These factors contribute even more to reflux at night when the enlarged abdominal wall or pregnant uterus press on the stomach.

In addition to weight, dietary issues, alcohol consumption, and anatomic factors, other medical conditions or medications for other problems can also lead to GERD symptoms. As they age, people tend to take more medications, and many medications can affect stomach acid production, the speed at which the stomach empties, and the ability of the LES to maintain its strength. High blood pressure medications called calcium channel blockers, such as nifedipine, can relax the LES. Drugs used for depression such as tricyclic antidepressants and drugs for psychosis impair stomach emptying.

We have tried to touch on a few of the reasons that people may develop new-onset GERD. However, people can experience reflux for a variety of reasons. It is important that you read through the remainder of this book and find the specific areas that may interest you to help explain your GERD.

## 12. How can I improve my symptoms of GERD?

The best way to minimize and possibly avoid GERD is to eliminate or reduce the factors that are within your control. Simple changes to make to start include lifestyle choices.

Immediately after you eat something, your body produces the greatest amount of acid for digestion of that food. Anytime you lie flat stomach acids can reflux into the esophagus. To reduce GERD symptoms, avoid eating late at night or wait at least 2 hours after you eat before you lie down. By coordinating your sleep habits and eating habits, you can allow ample time for the acid and food to pass through the stomach and can minimize reflux.

*To reduce GERD symptoms, avoid eating late at night or wait at least 2 hours after you eat before you lie down.*

21

A simple maneuver to improve nighttime GERD is to elevate the head of your bed. You can do this simply by placing small wooden blocks or bricks under the head of your bed. You can elevate your head by using special pillows called "Wedgies," which are available at surgical supply stores. This type of pillow allows your head and chest to be elevated at an incline, which helps keep your stomach below the level of your esophagus. Another nighttime tactic to try is to sleep on your left side. This position moves the stomach below the level of the esophagus and helps bring gravity back into the equation.

Certain foods and the way you eat your meals can also exacerbate GERD. Spicy, acidic, citrus, tomato-based, fatty, and fried foods can aggravate GERD symptoms. Some of these foods promote the production of more stomach acid, whereas others delay the stomach from emptying because they require more time for digestion to complete. By avoiding these types of foods, you can decrease the likelihood of GERD.

Other types of foods, such as alcohol, chocolate, or peppermint, can also cause reflux by relaxing the LES, which lowers its pressure. Normally, the LES acts as a one-way valve that relaxes to open during a swallow but stays contracted between swallows as a barrier to reflux. Avoiding foods that relax the LES can reduce the occurrence of reflux.

Caffeinated and carbonated beverages are also known to cause problems with reflux. The carbonation and gas in them can increase the pressure in the stomach and lead to heartburn. Also, carbonated drinks are acidic and can be irritating to an inflamed esophagus. Limiting these types of beverages can improve reflux.

Being overweight and eating large meals are closely related to GERD. Both of these factors can cause increased pressure in the stomach that can lead to reflux. Extra body weight in the abdomen increases pressure on the stomach and can force acid back into the esophagus. When you eat large meals, you overfill your stomach, which not only increases pressure in the stomach but slows stomach emptying and promotes GERD. Eating smaller meals will not only help people control their weight, but also helps reduce reflux symptoms.

Other lifestyle changes that may also be beneficial include stopping smoking, losing weight, and wearing loose clothing. Smoking hinders the protective factors against reflux, for example, decreasing saliva production. Wearing loose clothing and losing weight reduce the pressure on the stomach that can cause acidic fluid to be forced back into the esophagus.

These are only a few suggestions to help you improve your symptoms of GERD. As you read through the book, you'll notice many other lifestyle changes you can make to help reduce reflux symptoms.

Richard's comment:

*Over the years I have come to the realization that if I have a large, late meal, I will have acid reflux during the night. Also, a pepperoni pizza will spark an incident and a very uncomfortable evening.*

# PART TWO

# Symptoms and Atypical Manifestations of GERD

How do I know whether my heart is causing the chest pain?

Is there a difference between daytime and nighttime GERD?

What are alarm signs of GERD?

*More...*

## 13. How do I know whether my heart is causing the chest pain?

Heartburn is a pain in the chest, but is a type of misnomer. True heartburn is related to refluxing acidic materials back into the esophagus where is passes through the chest, which causes a burning sensation. Even though the name is heartburn, the condition actually has nothing to do with your heart's health. The name of this condition likely was developed when people mistakenly confused reflux pain with a heart attack.

A heart attack is a condition in which the heart receives a decreased amount of blood as a result of blockages or other reasons that cause decreased blood flow. The heart is a muscle, and when it doesn't receive enough blood, it can't pump normally and can become injured. Inadequate blood flow to the heart also causes discomfort or what people term *chest pain*. The chest pain occurs on the left side of the chest or behind the sternum, which is the breastbone in the center of your chest. But behind the sternum and the heart lies another organ, the esophagus, where it connects the mouth and the stomach.

*Reflux can be painful and dangerous over time, but heart pain sometimes called angina can be fatal.*

For this reason, the pain caused by reflux also causes "chest pain" and is sometimes confused with the pain associated with the heart. The pain can be very similar in quality, but it has drastically different consequences. Reflux can be painful and dangerous over time, but heart pain (sometimes called angina) can be fatal.

These two types of pain occur at different times, which can give you clues as to the source of the pain. Angina, heart-derived chest pain, or heart attacks usually occur after the heart has been stressed. It can occur after periods of exertion, for example, after running, walking long distances, swimming, or shoveling snow. The pain is usually associated with nausea, profuse sweating, and maybe even a feeling of lightheadedness. This type of pain can travel to the arm or jaw and may cause numbness or tingling. Angina may decrease after a period of rest, but it is usually not responsive to other remedies such as antacids.

On the other hand, reflux chest pain commonly feels like a burning sensation that usually occurs after you eat a meal. This pain stays in the chest area and can change if you change your position, depending on where the acid is refluxed. This type of pain may respond quickly to remedies such as antacids.

As you can see, these are two different types of pain that have very different qualities and consequences. The typical differences are not always as clear as mentioned here, as with anything in life. The two types of pain can almost blend into one another, so it is important to seek out the cause of chest pain to make sure you are not putting yourself at danger by leaving a heart problem unattended.

## 14. What about other chest symptoms with GERD?

GERD can affect other systems in your chest besides your mouth and stomach. To understand how it can affect other systems in your chest, it is important for you to visualize the anatomy of the human body.

*GERD can affect other systems in your chest besides your mouth and stomach.*

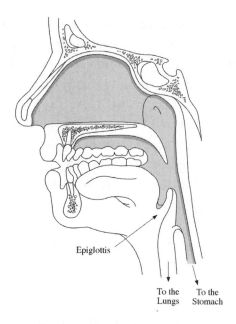

**Figure 6    Mouth and Nose.**

Visualize the path food takes as it moves through your body (see Figure 6). You can see that it moves to the back of the mouth and then makes a sharp turn down into the esophagus. Similarly, when you breathe through your nose, the air enters the nasal passages and follows a similar path down toward the lungs through the **trachea,** the windpipe. Where both the food and air take the sharp turn downward, they actually share the same channel in the back of your mouth, then this channel separates to conduct air to the lungs and food to the stomach. A valve called the epiglottis directs air and food to the correct place. Because food and air share the same passage, we are able to breathe through both our nose and mouth.

You might be wondering what breathing and the path the air takes have to do with reflux. The valve that controls the path of food and air is very thin, and the distance between the food pipe and the windpipe is also only a matter of a few millimeters. Because of the intimate relationship between the "airway" and the "food way," reflux can affect any part of the lungs or airway.

As the refluxed acid comes in contact with your airway, it can cause other symptoms in your chest, including persistent coughing and irritation of your throat, which causes some people to feel like they constantly have to clear their throats. The irritation can become so severe that it may even affect your voice box, which can cause you to have a hoarse voice. Finally, it is thought that people whose airways are constantly affected by acid reflux can develop hypersensitive airways and that this may eventually lead to asthma or make asthma worse, requiring more asthma medication.

## 15. Can I have chest pain caused by conditions other than GERD?

GERD is only one of the many conditions that can cause chest pain. Other causes of chest pain range from life-threatening to minor inconveniences. Of course, a severe and life-threatening cause of chest pain is a heart attack as discussed earlier (see Question 13).

For instance, a pulmonary embolism is a life-threatening condition that can cause severe chest pain. A pulmonary embolism is a blood clot that travels to the lungs and decreases blood flow to the lungs. It can lead to difficulty breathing and associated chest pain.

Another cause of chest pain is an aortic dissection, which occurs when the main blood vessel from the heart, the aorta, is affected and weak. The aorta can weaken with age, and it might keep expanding because of the blood pressure, which causes a tearing chest pain. In severe instances, the dissection can expand enough that it can burst. Both a pulmonary embolism and aortic dissection are fatal conditions unless emergency medical care is obtained.

A pneumothorax is an acute condition that causes chest pain and also requires immediate medical attention. A pneumothorax is a lung that "collapses" for any reason. This can lead to severe pain and difficulty breathing, and the lung should be reexpanded as quickly as possible.

Other more minor chest pain conditions include pericarditis, which is an inflammation of the lining of the heart that can be treated with medication. Also, some skin rashes can cause pain when they occur on the chest. Finally, the chest is made up of many muscles and bones. Costochondritis, or arthritis of the chest wall, can also produce chest pain.

These are only a few of the conditions that can mimic GERD. Please note that all of these conditions have serious risks and can be life-threatening. It might be difficult for you to identify the cause of your chest pain because the pain resulting from any of the conditions mentioned can be so similar at times. If you experience symptoms, see a doctor to look into the cause.

## 16. Can I have GERD without any symptoms?

Yes, GERD can occur with "silent" symptoms. Each individual's body reacts differently to different situations, so not everyone will have heartburn and be diagnosed with GERD. "Silent GERD" is one of the most difficult conditions to diagnose.

Instead of complaining of heartburn, often some people report sleep disruption, which is caused by acid refluxed into the esophagus as they lie down to sleep. As the acid travels up into the esophagus, people occasionally become aroused from their sleep. These sleep disturbances can occur regularly and cause severe interruptions to their sleep. Therefore, physicians should consider a diagnosis of GERD when people present with complaints of difficulty sleeping.

People with silent GERD also present with a persistent cough. As mentioned earlier, stomach acid may reflux up from the stomach into the esophagus and enter the trachea. This can lead to irritation of the airways and cause a cough and, in more severe instances, asthma attacks. Silent GERD can damage the voice box and cause voice changes such as hoarseness. An ear, nose, and throat (ENT) doctor can make this diagnosis by passing a tiny scope up the nose and down into the airway to examine the area. The ENT doctor can see changes caused by chronic acid damage, even in the absence of typical GERD symptoms. In fact, ENT doctors send many patients for further evaluation for GERD.

Finally, people may have ongoing reflux and not notice it if it remains silent. Over time, the acid refluxing up from the stomach can cause damage to the throat and eventually to the mouth. Throat damage may not present as heartburn, but when damage occurs in the mouth, people tend to notice. People or their dentists may notice the dental erosions, which may be the first indication of silent GERD in some people.

*People with silent GERD also present with a persistent cough. As mentioned earlier, stomach acid may reflux up from the stomach into the esophagus and enter the trachea. This can lead to irritation of the airways.*

Richard's comment:

*If I have a bout with acid reflux during the night, I can be assured that the next day my voice is going to be very hoarse. This probably is caused by the acid that is regurgitated during the night that makes me feel like I am drowning.*

## 17. Can GERD manifest as mouth symptoms in the absence of typical chest discomfort?

Yes, mouth symptoms can occur in the absence of chest discomfort. The acid can travel up from the stomach through the esophagus and into your mouth; this is called regurgitation. Most individuals experience symptoms with acid reflux; however, this is not always the case. Occasionally, people may not feel any pain because their esophagus has a decreased sensation to pain, or over the years they have become accustomed to the feeling and might not even notice it. This is called silent reflux. Without these people knowing it, the acid is traveling up into their mouths and causing different types of symptoms.

When acid enters the mouth, it brings with it some of the contents of the stomach, such as partially digested food, stomach enzymes, and acid that can leave a sour and bitter taste. If regurgitation occurs often, people can develop bad breath or dental problems. Acid regurgitation can cause cavities or can damage tooth enamel which results in discoloration of the teeth. However, before you attribute bad breath to GERD, have a dentist check to ensure that no cavities could be causing the bad breath.

As acid makes it way up to your mouth, your body reacts by producing saliva to try to neutralize the acid. The acid mixed with the excessive saliva can create a pasty, thick residue sometimes called *water brash* in your mouth.

As you can see, the symptoms in your mouth (e.g., bad breath, pasty saliva) can be very different from the painful symptoms such as heartburn in your chest.

## 18. Is there a difference between daytime and nighttime GERD?

GERD can occur at any time because the stomach is constantly producing acid, but acid production varies at different times. Food enters the mouth and moves down to the stomach, stimulating production of stomach enzymes and acid for digestion. The first major step in food processing is in the stomach, which slowly moves material into the small intestines where nutrients are absorbed. Certain fried and high-fat foods can stimulate the stomach to produce more acid and digestive juices than normal. Also, fatty foods slow stomach emptying, which means acidic material sits in the stomach for longer periods of time. Both of these factors explain why GERD symptoms might increase after you eat larger and fatty meals.

Nighttime GERD occurs because when you lie down to sleep, your stomach is actually level with or higher than your esophagus. This allows stomach fluid and acid to flow into the esophagus. Because of nighttime reflux, you might experience sleeping difficulties, wake up frequently, and be tired the next day.

*As you can see, the symptoms in your mouth (e.g., bad breath, pasty saliva) can be very different from the painful symptoms such as heartburn in your chest.*

*Nighttime GERD occurs because when you lie down to sleep, your stomach is actually level with or higher than your esophagus.*

In some ways, nocturnal GERD can actually be more dangerous than daytime GERD is. During the day, we subconsciously swallow, frequently clearing acid from the esophagus. While sleeping, we do not spontaneously swallow and so acid is not frequently cleared from the esophagus. Therefore, acid that flows back into the esophagus can sit there for extended periods of time and cause damage to the esophageal lining.

*Nighttime reflux is also worse because while sleeping you do not have the ability to protect your airway as you do when you are awake during the day.*

Nighttime reflux is also worse because while sleeping you do not have the ability to protect your airway as you do when you are awake during the day. If you have food or fluid in your mouth, while you're awake you can swallow it properly and can keep it out of your lungs. If you regurgitate while you're asleep, you can easily inhale fluid into your lungs. This can result in voice changes, chronic cough, chronic throat clearing, asthma, or pneumonia.

Management and prevention of day versus night symptoms are different. During the day, restrict your intake of certain foods such as caffeine, mint, spices, tomato, and citrus-based foods. At night, be sure not to eat for at least two hours prior to bedtime to reduce reflux symptoms. The major difference between day and night GERD management is in your body position. During the day, normally you are upright, but when you lie down at night, you reduce the protective effects of gravity. At night, you can use gravity to your advantage by elevating your esophagus over your stomach. Put bricks or cinderblocks under the legs at the head of your bed or use a wedge pillow to elevate your chest and head. Try sleeping with your left side down to help restore the benefits of gravity and improve symptoms.

Richard's comment:

*I have not experienced acid reflux during the day; in fact my days are usually very comfortable. But if daytime GERD is anything like the nasty nighttime GERD I suffer, then I'm very fortunate not to have both.*

## 19. Can GERD cause changes in my voice?

Yes, GERD can cause changes in your voice. High reflux can irritate your voice box, or **larynx**. Chronic acid damage of the larynx can cause voice changes. Repeated acid damage of the voice box can cause growths (polyps) to develop and can increase your risk of cancer. Cancer of the larynx is the most common cancer of the head and neck and is usually related to smoking. However, laryngeal cancer has been reported in people who have never smoked and who do not live with a smoker. These people might have developed cancer of the larynx as a result of acid reflux.

*High reflux can irritate your voice box or **larynx**.*

## 20. What are alarm signs of GERD?

GERD can cause many symptoms. When symptoms start affecting your overall health, you should seek medical attention. Look for the following key signs to distinguish the severity of your GERD:

- Do you experience GERD or heartburn 3 or more times per week?
- Is the pain in your chest from heartburn or reflux debilitating?
- Does the pain radiate to your arm or cause you to become short of breath?
- Does the pain wake you from sleep or prevent you from getting a full night's rest?

*When symptoms start affecting your overall health, you should seek medical attention.*

- Have these symptoms been ongoing for more than 6 months?
- Do you have a persistent and unexplained cough?
- Is your asthma difficult to control with conventional medications?
- Has the reflux caused you to lose weight over the past few months?
- Do you have pain after you eat?
- Have you tried **over-the-counter medications** but find they are no longer working?
- Do you have any difficulty swallowing?
- Do you wake up from sleep coughing, choking, or short of breath?
- Do you have unexplained repeated episodes of bronchitis or pneumonia?

People may ignore the symptoms and let them persist for a while, but reflux can damage your body. If you answered yes to any of the preceding questions, these signs should prompt you to seek medical attention and see your doctor.

# PART THREE

# Hiatal Hernias, the Lower Esophageal Sphincter, and Reflux

What do the lower esophageal sphincter (LES) and stomach have to do with reflux?

What is a hiatal hernia and why does it cause reflux?

Will my hiatal hernia get worse, and what are the complications?

*More ...*

## 21. What do the lower esophageal sphincter (LES) and stomach have to do with reflux?

Reflux occurs when acid and stomach enzymes are able to move in the wrong direction through the lower esophageal sphincter back into the esophagus.

Normally, the LES is a one-way valve and only allows food to pass from the esophagus to the stomach. However, when people suffer from reflux, the LES does not function properly and acid and stomach enzymes can travel up into the esophagus. At rest, the LES is closed and relaxes, opening during a swallow. Inappropriate relaxation or weakness of the LES as occurs with a hiatal hernia is a major cause of reflux.

## 22. What is a hiatal hernia and why does it cause reflux?

Normally, a muscle called the diaphragm separates the abdomen and chest. The diaphragm is the main muscle that controls breathing. The esophagus passes from the back of the throat into the chest, behind the heart, down through a hole in the diaphragm called a hiatus to join with the stomach in the abdomen. The position of the stomach and the esophagus as it passes through the diaphragm are important and are maintained by ligaments that hold the structures in proper position.

As you age, the ligaments holding the stomach in place can stretch, and the hiatus in the diaphragm can enlarge. The result is that part of the stomach can move abnormally into the chest, creating a condition known as a hiatal or hiatus hernia. Normal position of the junction of the esophagus and stomach is required to maintain appropriate strength of the lower esophageal sphincter, a muscle within the wall of the esophagus. The LES is the main barrier to stomach acid reflux. When a hiatal hernia occurs, the LES becomes weaker, predisposing you to reflux.

There are two major types of hiatal hernias, and both increase GERD. Typically, people refer to a **sliding hiatal hernia**. It is called a *sliding* type because the stomach can slide in and out of the chest. The other type of hiatal hernia is called a **paraesophageal hernia**. A paraesophageal hernia is a condition in which the stomach slides up into the chest through the hiatus alongside the esophagus. Paraesophageal hernias are more common in those older than 70 years. In a paraesophageal hernia, the stomach is in the chest though its blood supply comes through the diaphragm from the abdomen. The blood supply can be interrupted if the blood vessels twist. Temporary interruption of blood flow can cause nausea, vomiting, and pain. In severe cases, part of the stomach can die off, accompanied by bleeding, pain, and, if untreated, death. For this reason, if you have a paraesophageal hernia, get a referral to a surgeon to have it repaired.

*Normal position of the junction of the esophagus and stomach is required to maintain appropriate strength of the lower esophageal sphincter, a muscle within the wall of the esophagus.*

**Sliding hiatal hernia**

the most common type of hiatal hernia in which part of the stomach slides from the abdomen into the chest.

## 23. What are the symptoms of a hiatal hernia?

A hiatal hernia does not cause pain. Symptoms you might experience are heartburn and regurgitation. A hiatal hernia causes the LES to be less effective, resulting in GERD, but the hiatal hernia itself really has no symptoms. Many patients report dyspepsia, which is the feeling of a "sour stomach," and they think that means they have a hiatal hernia. But dyspepsia is a nonspecific stomach disorder treated with a proton pump inhibitor (PPI).

## 24. Will my hiatal hernia get worse, and what are the complications?

*The chance of developing a hiatal hernia increases with age.*

The chance of developing a hiatal hernia increases with age. Complications of a sliding hiatal hernia are ulcers with possible bleeding. Frequently, patients are referred for evaluation for anemia. **Anemia** is a low blood count and is from either blood loss or inadequate blood production. Low iron stores in the body frequently cause anemia because iron is required to make red blood cells. The initial evaluation for iron deficiency anemia is a colonoscopy to rule out a bleeding cancer. A small amount of long-standing bleeding depletes iron stores. Once a colon-bleeding source has been eliminated, an upper endoscopy test is done. This can show whether a large sliding hiatal hernia contains ulcers that bleed chronically. Very rarely, a cancer can form in a hiatal hernia and can bleed chronically, resulting in anemia.

# PART FOUR

# *Lifestyle, Medications, Diet, and GERD*

Can medicines exacerbate GERD?

Will eating fast food make my GERD worse?

Can my weight affect my GERD?

*More...*

## 25. Can stress increase GERD symptoms?

Stress affects all people differently. Each individual's body reacts differently to stress, whether it comes in the form of a new assignment at work or a stressful conversation at home. Stress incorporates itself into your life and must be dealt with daily. If stress always led to GERD, most people would experience heartburn and reflux almost every day! But this is not the case.

In stressful situations, your body responds by producing hormones that regulate organ function. During times of stress, the colon, for example, responds by contracting and emptying itself. This can cause you to experience diarrhea in times of stress. Others may experience a flushed feeling or warmth in their face.

Some people do experience heartburn in times of stress. This can occur because stress hormones cause stomach relaxation, and food can linger in the stomach for increased periods of time. Stress hormones may increase stomach acid production. Both of these stress-related factors may result in flares of GERD during emotionally difficult times.

Stress can also lead to other symptoms that are similar to a flare of GERD. Stress hormones affect the heart, increasing its workload, and also may increase blood pressure. Some people can feel angina, a type of pain related to the heart, which is increased in times of stress. This can often be confused with GERD because of its location in the chest. As mentioned previously,

*In stressful situations, your body responds by producing hormones that regulate organ function.*

heart pain and reflux pain are very similar and are difficult at times to distinguish from each other.

Each person has a different threshold for stress, and different events are stressful to each individual. However, in times of severe stress, hormones can cause reflux or other symptoms of GERD.

## 26. Can smoking cause GERD?

Smoking is a dangerous habit that can result in many health risks. Smoking is associated with many cancers, heart disease, vascular disease, stomach ulcers, and lung disease, to name a few. Some studies have shown a link between smoking and GERD. Even though smoking does not directly cause GERD, it can exacerbate GERD symptoms.

The nicotine in cigarette smoke can reduce the ability of the lower esophageal sphincter to contract or close, allowing acid to reflux. The LES is a muscle that keeps acid produced in the stomach from entering the esophagus. Anything that relaxes this muscle (cigarettes, alcohol, foods, or medications) causes the esophagus to be exposed to acid. Studies have shown that smoking increases irritation of the esophagus when acid refluxes and increases symptoms of heartburn. Aside from discomfort caused by reflux, the greatest complication of GERD is the development of cancer, and smoking greatly increases esophageal cancer risk.

*The nicotine in cigarette smoke can reduce the ability of the lower esophageal sphincter to contract or close, allowing acid to reflux.*

Cigarette smoke, particularly nicotine, can dry out your mouth, which decreases saliva production. You swallow saliva constantly, and this aids digestion of food and lubricates the esophagus. Saliva neutralizes acid and is protective when stomach acid refluxes into esophagus by helping to clear it.

Some people are in the habit of reaching for a cigarette right after a meal, which can exacerbate problems. After you eat, the stomach produces acid for digestion. Then, if you smoke, nicotine and cigarette smoke enter the bloodstream and impair contraction of the LES. The relaxed LES and a plentiful supply of acid are set up for GERD to occur. So, in this way, even though smoking may not directly cause GERD, it can make GERD worse.

## 27. Can medicines exacerbate GERD?

Most medications are taken by mouth; they are absorbed through the gut and then enter the blood-stream. From the bloodstream, medications can act on various organs. All medications have desired actions and possible side effects. Sometimes when a medicine is prescribed for one problem, it can end up leading to another problem. Every individual's body can react differently to various medications, and it is not always possible to predict drug effects and side effects.

*Some medications can exacerbate GERD.*

Some medications can exacerbate GERD. Good examples are certain blood pressure drugs. Antihypertensive medications, or medications for high blood pressure, are of many types and have multiple mechanisms of action to effect lower blood pressure. One class of such drugs is called calcium-channel blockers, and they are quite effective at lowering blood pressure. But, as mentioned, all medications can have side effects that are generally undesirable. Calcium-channel blockers relax a type of muscle cell in the body called smooth muscle; hormones and other local factors control these muscle cells. Smooth muscle is a muscle type that is not within your conscious control, unlike the muscles in your arms or legs. Smooth muscles line blood vessels, and when these muscles are relaxed, your blood pressure drops. Smooth muscle also lines the gut, including the esophagus, the lower esophageal sphincter, and the colon (large intestine). Side effects of calcium channel blockers are relaxation of the LES, which can lead to reflux, and relaxation of the colon, which can lead to constipation.

Many medications are directly toxic to the esophagus and damage the lining of the esophagus. Examples of these are aspirin and over-the-counter pain medications, some antibiotics, some minerals such as potassium and iron, and drugs for osteoporosis such as alendronate sodium (Fosamax). These drugs are either acidic or caustic, and manufacturers generally recommend that they be taken with a lot of water or with food. People who take drugs for osteoporosis should remain upright for 30 minutes after taking the pills. This is suggested so that the pill does not sit in the esophagus and dissolve, which would allow it to damage the lining of the esophagus. Staying upright helps the pill move down into the stomach.

*Many medications are directly toxic to the esophagus and damage the lining of the esophagus.*

These are only a few examples of drugs that can affect the esophagus. Medications can cause problems with GERD for a variety of different reasons; the three main reasons are as follows:

- The medication relaxes the LES and allows acid to reflux back into the esophagus.

- The medication irritates and directly damages the lining of the esophagus, which can increase the damage caused by reflux.
- The medication can cause the body's digestive system to slow down, which leads to food lingering in and more acid production in the stomach.

## 28. Which specific medications can exacerbate GERD or damage the esophagus?

As mentioned, medications can act in different ways to affect GERD and reflux symptoms (see Table 1). Medications can either affect the nerves that control the LES or the muscles that control the tightness of the LES.

*Medications can either affect the nerves that control the LES or the muscles that control the tightness of the LES.*

All muscles, including the LES, are controlled by nerves. Muscles of the gut are called smooth muscle and you cannot consciously control them by thinking about it. The nerves transmit signals from the brain to the rest of the body. Nerves that make up what is called the autonomic nervous system automatically control the LES muscle cells. The autonomic nervous system controls functions that are essential for living, such as breathing, contraction of the heart muscle, food digestion, and blood flow throughout the body. For this reason, if medication can affect smooth muscle or the nerves that control the smooth muscle, then it can affect gut function.

The different classes of medications to be aware of include medications for depression (antidepressants), high blood pressure medications (beta-blockers, calcium channel blockers, and nitrates), antinausea

**Table 1   Medications that May Cause Reflux or Heartburn**

| Medication (generic) | Medication (trade) | Uses |
|---|---|---|
| Amitriptyline | Elavil | Antidepressant medication |
| Diazepam | Valium | Antianxiety |
| Diltiazem | Cardizem, Cartia, Tiazac | Calcium channel blocker—High blood pressure |
| Doxepin | Sinequan | Antidepressant medication |
| Felodipine | Plendil | Calcium channel blocker—High blood pressure |
| Imipramine | Tofranil | Antidepressant medication |
| Isosorbide nitrate | Imdur, Nitrodur | Nitrates—High blood pressure or angina |
| Labetalol | n/a | Beta-Blocker—High blood pressure |
| Levodopa | Sinemet | Anti-Parkinsons |
| Nifedipine | Adalat, Procardia | Calcium channel blocker - High blood pressure |
| Nortriptyline | Aventyl, Pamelor | Antidepressant medication |
| Progestin | n/a | Birth control or abnormal menstrual bleeding |
| Theophylline | Theolair, Uniphyl | AntiAsthma |
| Metoprolol | Toprol | Beta blocker—High blood pressure |

medications (anticholinergics), pain medications (narcotics), hormones, sedatives, and some asthma medications (theophylline).

The anticholinergic medications, such as antinausea medications, control the autonomic nerves responsible for digestion. These medications can decrease the nerve output to the muscles of the LES, thereby causing the muscles to relax and worsening the symptoms of GERD. Anticholingeric medications also slow stomach emptying, giving reflux more time to occur. Examples of commonly prescribed anticholinergic medications used for nausea are prochlorperazine (Compazine), promethazine (Phenergan), and scopolamine.

Medications for high blood pressure called calcium-channel blockers or beta-blockers can, on the other hand, directly affect the tightness of the muscles of the LES. These medications affect certain muscles in the blood vessels and relax them to lower blood pressure. Because they relax smooth muscle, they delay stomach emptying. Examples of these are nifedipine (Procardia), diltiazem (Cartia and Cardizem), verapamil (Calan), inderal (Propanolol), and nadolol (Corgard).

Medications for asthma can also affect the LES and impair its ability to contract. An example is theo-phylline, which relaxes smooth muscle. Smooth muscle lines the airways of the lungs. When these muscles go into spasms, asthma occurs. Asthma medications work by relaxing and opening the airways to make breathing easier. However, these muscles are similar to the muscles controlling the LES. Therefore, along with relaxing the muscles in the lungs, asthma medications can also relax the muscle in the LES. Asthma medications that can exacerbate reflux include theophylline (Uniphyl) and some inhalers such as albuterol.

Through similar mechanisms, other medications, including pain medications, sedating medications, and even antidepressants, can also loosen the LES and cause reflux symptoms to worsen. Many medications used for depression have anticholinergic effects (similar to medications for nausea); examples are amitriptyline (Elavil), desipramine, and imipramine. Narcotics used for severe pain such as morphine, fentanyl, long-acting narcotics oxycodone (Oxycontin), and morphine sulphate (MS Contin) all delay **gastric** emptying. Female hormones also relax the LES; these include most estrogen-containing medications and are commonly used by women going through menopause.

Finally, as mentioned previously, most medications used for thinning of the bones or osteoporosis are direct irritants and can damage the esophagus. This class of drugs is called bisphosphonates and limits the body's ability to metabolize bone. This limits breakdown of bones and keeps them strong. These medications should not be taken by people who have difficulty swallowing because the pills can lodge in the esophagus, causing damage. An example of bisphosphonate medication is alendronate (Fosamax). Several other medications are also acidic or corrosive and damage the esophagus on contact. These are potassium pills, iron supplements, quinidine (a heart medication) and antibiotics such as tetracycline and doxycycline.

All of these medications are very commonly used and have the potential side effect of increasing GERD or directly damaging the esophagus.

## 29. Which medications can affect both esophagus and stomach?

The esophagus and stomach are exposed to a wide variety of consumed substances that are potentially irritating or damaging. For this reason, a protective layer of cells called the **mucosa** lines the stomach and esophagus. The mucosa is a microscopic layer of cells, like skin that it is constantly changing and renewing itself. In the esophagus, the mucosa is a smooth surface that is slippery and allows substances swallowed to pass easily through to the stomach. Stomach mucosa is different; it has both a protective function and it produces and secretes material. The lining of the stomach produces acid and some enzymes used for digestion, and it protects the stomach from the acid it contains. Stomach acid is so strong it can remove paint from a car. Despite the durable protective nature of stomach and esophageal mucosa, they are still subject to damage by certain medications.

The problem arises when the esophagus and stomach are not able to keep up with the constant injury to their linings. Some medications affect the mucosa so much that the body cannot produce cells fast enough and certain areas become exposed, allowing damage from acid or other digestive juices. Medications that can cause this type of injury include certain antibiotics, medications for osteoporosis, and even simple over-the-counter pain medications. These medications can cause problems by increasing acid production, which irritates the esophagus and stomach.

Antibiotics from a drug class called macrolides, which includes erythromycin, azithromycin (Zithro-

**Mucosa**

the lining of the gut. Each gut organ has a special mucosa that can be identified under the microscope. The mucosa is like the "skin" lining the gut.

*Some medications affect the mucosa so much that the body cannot produce cells fast enough and certain areas become exposed, allowing damage from acid or other digestive juices.*

max), and clarithromycin (Biaxin), can cause stomach irritation. Medications for osteoporosis, the bisphosphonates, can cause problems by irritating the lining of the esophagus as well as that of the stomach. Bisphosphonates, which include risendronate (Actonel) and alendronate, can directly affect the lining of the esophagus and increase the acid production in the stomach. Finally, pain medications related to aspirin in the drug family called **nonsteroidal anti-inflammatory drugs (NSAIDs)**, which includes over-the-counter medication such as naproxen (Aleve) and ibuprofen (Advil and Motrin), can irritate the stomach lining and cause ulcers in the esophagus, stomach, or **duodenum**. Symptoms from these medications include heartburn, abdominal pain, and nausea.

## 30. How can I avoid GERD problems if I have to take my pills?

Any medication has side effects, and sometimes you might resort to alternative medications to alleviate particular side effects, but in some cases you may not have a choice but to take a drug that will exacerbate your GERD. Many of the medications mentioned earlier are necessary to treat medical conditions, and the side effects that come along with them may be unavoidable. However, even if the side effects are present, you may be able to take precautions to decrease their severity. It is important to remember that if a medication has side effects, there may be an alternate way to take the medication or there may be an alternative drug to use for the same condition. The disease should always be worse than the cure! It is important to read the labels on medications, and if you have questions or problems with side effects, you should discuss them with your pharmacist. If the problems are beyond the control of the pharmacist, you should contact the doctor who prescribed the medications to check into possible alternatives.

*It is important to take medications as directed.*

It is important to take medications as directed. Many medications are specified to be taken with food to limit side effects. However, some need to be taken hours before or after eating because foods can interfere with drug absorption and action. The most important thing you can do is read the label.

Remember that the longer these medications are in contact with the esophagus or stomach lining, the more damage they potentially can do. Once you put them in your mouth and swallow, it is important to use gravity to your advantage. Medications known to irritate the esophagus should be taken while you are sitting or standing up. Once you have taken the pill, it is important that you do not immediately lie down. By lying down, you put the stomach at the same level or above the level of the esophagus, which can allow the pill and even the stomach acid to reflux into the esophagus.

*It is very important to take enough water with medications.*

It is very important to take enough water with medications. Water helps move the pills from the esophagus to the stomach by lubricating the esophagus so as to provide a slippery surface for the pills to easily pass down the esophagus and avoid damaging the lining.

Commonly, people take medications dry or with a tiny sip of water, and then go to sleep for the night. This increases the chances the pill will stick in the esophagus all night, causing damage. When we do an endoscopy test, we commonly find a problem called a pill ulcer. Classically, this is caused when you take an aspirin or ibuprofen at bedtime without drinking enough water. The pill then sits in your esophagus all night, burning a hole in the lining, which results in an ulcer. Pill ulcers cause severe pain when you swallow. Thankfully, these are easily avoided and generally heal after a few days.

Finally, it is important to note whether the medication has a protective coating that may help avoid damage to your esophagus and your stomach. If this is the case, do not chew the pills. These protective coatings (sometimes called **enteric coating**) can allow the pill to pass through the esophagus and stomach, hopefully doing as little damage as possible, before it is digested in the small intestine.

By using all these measures, you can avoid the major problems related to reflux caused by medications. However, this is not a guarantee that you will avoid side effects. If you have questions or problems, contact your pharmacist or doctor.

Richard's comment:

*I have a heart condition that requires me to take a daily beta-blocker and aspirin to thin my blood. I have not noticed the beta-blocker causing me discomfort, but the aspirin irritated my stomach. When I switched to an enteric aspirin, that symptom disappeared. I also use plenty of water in taking my pills to make sure they get to my stomach without sticking in my throat.*

## 31. Can exercise affect my reflux?

Exercise is generally good and beneficial, but not always. Exercise is good for improving strength, heart conditioning, weight control, and overall health. On the other hand, it can affect reflux and make it worse. Exercise can cause problems with reflux because of its effects on the digestive system and the physical positioning and pressures it places on the stomach and the esophagus. However, acid reflux should not be a reason to avoid exercising because exercise has so many positive and beneficial effects on your body. Exercising properly can help you avoid the problems caused by reflux disease.

When people engage in physical activity, the body shunts blood away from the stomach to the muscles that are being used in exercise. This diversion of blood makes the stomach and small intestine work less efficiently and requires that food remain in the stomach longer for proper digestion. The longer the food remains in the stomach, the more acid can build up and the more reflux potential is created by the body.

You have heard people say it is important to wait one hour after eating before you go swimming or exercise. There is some truth to this. As you participate in physical activity the food and all the contents of your stomach slosh around. A stomachful of sloshing food and acid can also move up into the esophagus and cause severe reflux. For this reason, it is important to eat smaller meals before exercising and allow ample time for the food to be digested before you participate in intense exercise and activity.

The types of food you eat around the time of exercise can also make a difference. Foods that are higher in fat content generally take longer to digest and remain in the stomach a longer period of time. These foods also require higher acid production for complete digestion, which is a good setup for worsening reflux disease. Carbohydrates are digested more quickly and can pass through the stomach much easier, causing less reflux symptoms if you are going to exercise or participate in high-energy activity. Also, citrus and tomato-based foods, caffeine, mints, and chocolate all are associated with GERD.

While exercising, it is important that you replace fluid lost through sweating and perspiration by drinking liquids. Liquids are beneficial in that they help hydrate your body and move digested food through your digestive system. Certain liquids should, however, be avoided during exercise because they may increase reflux. Sodas and citrus juices are acidic and may have carbonation that promotes reflux. Caffeinated beverages relax the LES, facilitating reflux.

Finally, it is important to remember what type of exercise your body will be able to handle if you have bad reflux disease. Some exercises that involve bending over or into a hunched position, such as sit-ups, place extra pressure on the stomach, which may worsen reflux. Other activities, like swimming, in which the body is horizontal, can also cause problems when the stomach is level with or above the level of the esophagus.

However, the benefits of exercising far outweigh the dangers. Exercise can help vitalize so many organs in your body and can even help you lose weight, which can reduce the pressure on your stomach and improve reflux. So, don't try to avoid exercise, but rather modify the foods you eat before exercising, the timing of meals, and the activity so that exercise will not affect your reflux.

Richard's comment:

*When I have a reasonable dinner early in the evening and then take a 30- to 45-minute walk, my acid reflux symptoms are almost always nonexistent for the evening. The walking seems to calm my stomach and helps in the digestive process.*

## 32. What kind of foods can make GERD worse?

*Different types of food can increase reflux or can increase the amount of acid the stomach produces. These include high-fat foods, spicy foods, carbonated beverages, chocolate, mint, and alcohol.*

Different types of food can increase reflux or can increase the amount of acid the stomach produces. These include high-fat foods, spicy foods, carbonated beverages, chocolate, mint, and alcohol.

High-fat foods are more difficult to digest. The digestion of fatty food can cause increased stomach acid production and delays stomach emptying. Both of these effects cause higher amounts of acid to be present, and the longer time the food dwells in your stomach, the chances of reflux disease increase. Similarly, spicy foods can also increase acid production. Many people find that spicy foods are associated with symptoms of heartburn and reflux.

Alcoholic beverages can affect reflux symptoms in two ways. First, alcohol is an irritant to the esophageal mucosa and cause direct damage to it. Second, alcohol is a depressant, meaning it calms and relaxes you. Part of this action is the relaxation of muscles, including the lower esophageal sphincter. Both of these effects can result in increased reflux symptoms.

Carbonated beverages exacerbate reflux through multiple mechanisms. Many carbonated drinks, such as colas, contain caffeine that relaxes the LES. Further, the gas from carbonated drinks is released in the stomach. This excess gas causes belching; however, it also increases pressure within the stomach, facilitating GERD. Finally, all sodas are acidic and increase the overall amount of acid in the stomach, which can be highly corrosive. If you put a few drops of a commonly consumed cola on the hood of a car and let it sit overnight, the paint would begin peeling off by the next morning. Thankfully, foods in the gut do not sit in one place for long periods of time, which limits the amount of damage they can do.

Many foods cause relaxation of the LES, which increases GERD. Avoidance of these foods and drinks can help you control GERD and may eliminate or decrease your need for medications. In addition to those previously discussed, examples are citrus foods such as oranges, lemons, grapefruits, and limes; spicy foods; tomato-based foods and sauces; chocolate; mint; onions; and garlic. Some of these relax the LES, others increase gastric acid production. Avoid these foods particularly before going to sleep because sleeping slows stomach emptying. Tea or coffee with a chocolate cookie before bed is probably not a good idea for those with nocturnal GERD.

## 33. What kind of foods should I eat if I have GERD?

Question 32 discusses the foods you should avoid. Eating smaller meals should be your goal because they are emptied from the stomach faster and do not increase pressures within the stomach like a large meal does. Smaller and lighter meals can also help with weight control.

Most fruits and vegetables are preferred because they are healthy, low in fat, empty from the stomach relatively quickly, and are lower in acid. Some may actually settle your stomach.

On the other hand, juices such as orange, cranberry, grapefruit, tomato, and lemon can cause increased acid production in your stomach and lead to heartburn symptoms. If you do desire juices, seek out the low-acid alternatives that are available. Then, you can enjoy your share of juices and avoid the reflux symptoms associated with their full-acid counterparts.

Historically, before there were antiulcer medications such as H2 blockers or proton pump inhibitors, people with GERD followed a special diet called a "sippy diet." This diet worked for ulcers because it coated the stomach and neutralized acid. Unfortunately, in the new millennium, the sippy diet would not be recommended because it is very high in fat—but the concept was a good one. Foods and drinks were sipped constantly to neutralize acid as it was produced. Foods used in the sippy diet included creams, dairy products, cheeses, and eggs to name a few. Today there are low-fat alternative to these foods that are healthier and still help minimize stomach acid. Other foods that may be helpful for those with GERD are yogurts, soy products such as tofu, and low-fat cheeses. All of these are healthy, good for weight control, contain important necessary minerals such as calcium for bone health, and are great sources of protein.

Also, eating lean and low-fat meats are easier to digest and empty from the stomach faster. They are good sources of protein important for maintaining muscles, wound healing, and strength.

Finally, many sweets, liquors, and caffeinated beverages are also acid stimulating. The fat-free options of cookies and cakes are generally recommended. Liquors or alcohol should be avoided to maintain the LES pressure and prevent reflux symptoms. Also, caffeine-free teas and coffees stimulate less acid production and prevent heartburn.

Following these recommendations can help you control weight, limit LES relaxation and acid production, and improve overall health in addition to decreasing GERD.

## 34. Will eating fast food make my GERD worse?

Fast food is exactly what it sounds like: food that is available quickly with very little effort. Fast-food restaurants prepare foods that come ready made, have a long shelf life, are filling, are easy to make in vast quantities, and are cheap. They attract customers to return by making food very tasty, high in flavor, filling and "a good value for your dollar." Unfortunately, this is a very bad combination. Fast foods are very high in fat and are highly salted, and sodas are "liquid candy."

Overall, even though fast foods are presented as a good value, they really are not because they are unhealthy. Marketing of fast food has resulted in "super sizing" in an attempt to give you even more food for your money. The result is that two-thirds of all Americans are overweight, and one-third are **obese** (roughly 30 pounds overweight). The salt consumption and weight gain can result in high blood pressure, heart disease, and strokes. Super-sized drinks contain hundreds of calories of pure sugar and large amounts of caffeine. These are marketed to children, ensuring future fast-food consumers. This has caused an epidemic of overweight and obese children and an increase in diabetes occurring at younger ages.

*Super-sized drinks contain hundreds of calories of pure sugar and large amounts of caffeine.*

Most fast food is fried and high in fat, which makes it taste good. It is made of processed foods such as frozen meat patties and potatoes. Recent attention in the press has focused on the type of fat in fast food. Oils used for frying contain **"trans fat."** Trans fat improves food flavor and is inexpensive. Trans fat is likely the strongest contributor to heart disease, stroke and certain cancers in the American diet. It is recommended that trans fat be limited. There is very little green food other than a poor wilted leaf of lettuce virtually devoid of any nutritional value on a burger. These days, though, fast-food producers have realized that Americans are becoming smarter consumers and they have added fresh salads to their menus. Unfortunately, salads are topped with buttery croutons, high-fat cheeses, and fatty dressings, all contributing hundreds of calories and negating the beneficial effects of the salad. Other condiments are not benign, either. Ketchup is acidic and high in sugar; mayonnaise is very high in fat.

These large, fatty, and caffeinated meals increase GERD by impairing stomach emptying, increasing pressure within the stomach, and relaxing the LES. Because these foods are also available in most markets 24/7, people eat them at night before bed, increasing nighttime symptoms. Indirectly, these foods make people fatter, which is another precipitating cause or GERD. As a consequence of obesity, high blood pressure, heart disease, and diabetes, as a population Americans take more medications, which may have side effects that exacerbate GERD.

## 35. How else can I change my eating habits to prevent GERD?

Changing your lifestyle and eating habits is easier said than done. However, by making some simple modifications you can improve GERD symptoms and decrease some of the dangers associated with GERD.

As mentioned previously, eating late at night and eating large meals can increase your heartburn symptoms. If you lie down to sleep with a stomach full of food and acid, chances are you will experience heartburn symptoms. Avoiding late-night meals and avoiding eating for at least 2 hours prior to bedtime are good ways to start changing your lifestyle. Eating large meals increases reflux symptoms. By eating smaller meals rather than three large meals throughout the day, you can avoid putting pressure on the LES.

Changing the way you prepare foods can make a difference. Eat low-fat foods and prepare foods with a minimum of added calories to aid in maintaining a good weight. Broil or barbeque meats to avoid the addition of fat calories; lean meats, fish, and chicken are all good sources of protein. Avoid fatty or sugary condiments such as oils, mayonnaise, and ketchup to help cut calories. The easiest way to watch and reduce calories is by reading food labels and knowing the fat content. This is a good habit to get into and can benefit your health in the long run.

*For example, a 20-ounce cola, which is a regular-sized bottle, contains 250 calories and 65 grams of sugar—that is, 13 packets of sugar in one drink*

Breakfast cereals can contain large amounts of sugar. Salad dressings frequently are very high in fat, and low-fat alternatives are just as tasty. Low-fat milk and dairy products are a great source of protein and calcium. Sugar-free sodas are an easy and palatable choice and are comparable in taste to regular sugared sodas. For example, a 20-ounce cola, which is a regular-sized bottle, contains 250 calories and 65 grams of sugar—that is, 13 packets of sugar in one drink (and that is not even a super-sized one).

Dieting can be difficult, and by definition when you are dieting you are sacrificing or withholding something from yourself. Reading labels and educating yourself and understanding what you are eating enables you to make small, sensible changes that are easy, less painful, and maintainable in the long run. All of these strategies can help you lose weight and maintain it and control a major cause of GERD.

**Richard's comment:**

*My grandson asked one day, "Grampie, why don't you put dressing on your salad?" Over the years, I have come to realize that certain types of foods upset my stomach, whereas others have a settling effect. I try to live by the USDA food pyramid and really limit my sweets, condiments, and processed foods. The more I adhere to the USDA food pyramid, the better my stomach feels and the less acid reflux symptoms arise or incidences occur.*

## 36. Does GERD get worse with age?

Aging is inevitable and unavoidable; the body becomes less efficient at functioning and does not seem to "work like it used to." As you age, the tendency is that you will slowly gain weight, which contributes to GERD symptoms. Acid in the esophagus is neutralized by saliva, and saliva production decreases with age. Further, many medications used by the elderly cause dry mouth and decrease saliva production, compounding the problem. With increasing age, stomach emptying is slowed and further affected by medications.

Hiatal hernias, which promote GERD as a result of a loss of the normal function of the lower esophageal sphincter, become more common with age. A hiatal hernia occurs when the normal position of the anatomy and junction of the esophagus and stomach is lost (see Question 22). Ligaments that hold the stomach in its normal position become lax as you age. The diaphragm, the muscle that separates the chest from the abdomen, has a hole in it where the esophagus passes through to reach the stomach in the abdomen. This hole can enlarge with age,

*Hiatal hernias, which promote GERD as a result of a loss of the normal function of the lower esophageal sphincter, become more common with age.*

*It is important to recognize that with age, your body becomes more vulnerable to the dangers of acid reflux.*

enabling part of the stomach to enter the chest. The end result is a hiatal hernia.

It is important to recognize that with age, your body becomes more vulnerable to the dangers of acid reflux. With time, people are less mobile and less active; this can translate into more time spent in bed, where reflux risk is higher. Also with age, patients tend to take more medications, some of which can lead to reflux symptoms. These medications may cause direct damage to the esophagus, impair stomach emptying, decrease saliva production, cause ulcers, or relax the LES. The end result of these factors is an increase in reflux symptoms.

*Night symptoms include heartburn, regurgitation with coughing, choking, gasping for air, and a bitter taste in your mouth or excessive drooling.*

**Aspiration**

the process of food or liquid entering the airway or lungs. Aspiration can occur on swallowing and commonly happens in patients who have had prior strokes and who cannot swallow normally. Aspiration can also occur accompanying GERD. The refluxed material comes up through the esophagus to the mouth and then may be inhaled, damaging the airways (trachea or larynx) or lungs. Aspiration can result in severe pneumonias.

## 37. Does my bed make a difference in nighttime symptoms?

Your bed, its position, and type of mattress can make a difference in nighttime symptoms. As discussed previously, nighttime GERD can cause symptoms that you may not even be aware of. These symptoms can affect your sleep and make you wake up without feeling refreshed. Night symptoms include heartburn, regurgitation with coughing, choking, gasping for air, and a bitter taste in your mouth or excessive drooling. On rare occasions nocturnal regurgitation can lead to **aspiration** and pneumonia.

Nighttime reflux may not be related only to late meals and type of foods consumed but to the type of bed and the positioning of your bed. When you lie down, your stomach and esophagus are at the same level. This makes it easy for acid and stomach contents to flow back into the esophagus, causing reflux symptoms. The main strategy is to position yourself so that your esophagus and stomach are not at the same level, which can decrease the possibility of reflux and reduce nighttime symptoms. One way to raise the level of your head is to raise the entire head of the bed. Elevating the head of the bed can be achieved by placing risers or bricks underneath the feet of the bed to create an incline that keeps the esophagus at a higher level than your stomach. Wedge pillows also have the same effect; they are available at medical supply stores and will not affect your spouse or partner sharing your bed. Finally, a more expensive option is an adjustable bed, which allows elevation of the head of the bed. Any of these strategies will bring gravity back into the equation and help minimize nighttime acid reflux.

*Weight plays a major role in many aspects of your health and well-being.*

## 38. Can my weight affect my GERD?

Weight plays a major role in many aspects of your health and well-being. Being overweight can increase your chance of heart disease, diabetes, high blood pressure, strokes, certain cancers, and acid reflux. GERD has a higher association with those who are overweight as defined by an elevated body mass index.

**Body mass index (BMI)** is a standardized measure of weight for height. The BMI is calculated by taking your weight in kilograms and dividing it by your height in meters squared. For example, a woman 5 feet 2 inches who weighs 175 pounds has a BMI of 32 as compared to another woman who is 5 feet 8 inches and weighs 175 pounds with a BMI of 26. These women are the same weight, yet the shorter woman is considered obese and the taller woman is considered only mildly overweight. A BMI in the range of 18 to 25 is generally considered to be normal weight for height. A BMI of 25 to 30 is overweight, and a BMI greater than 30 is classified as obese. The BMI correlates to increasing risks of complications of obesity as the number increases. You can easily determine your BMI using various charts or by plugging your height and weight into the many programs available on personal digital assistants or the Internet.

Reflux is associated with increased weight or obesity for a number of reasons.

Extra abdominal weight creates more pressure on the stomach. In turn, this can lead to stomach contents and acid being forced up through the LES and can expose the esophagus to reflux symptoms. Some obese people tend to have poor eating habits that may include fast food or other high-calorie foods that promote GERD. Further, they may eat larger meals or snack prior to bed. Because many diseases are associated with being overweight, there is a tendency for obese people to take more medications, which can adversely impact reflux.

Given that multiple factors are at play in exacerbating reflux in those who are overweight, multiple issues can be acted on. Interestingly, only small changes in weight or minor modifications in eating habits can provide great benefits for reducing GERD.

## 39. When should I consider medications for GERD?

Initial management of GERD takes the form of lifestyle modification. Often, making small changes in diet or time of eating can improve symptoms. On the other hand, when you suffer from GERD and have tried the recommendations outlined in this book to no avail, medications may be in order.

Different types of medications and different tiers, or strengths, of medications are available for the treatment of GERD. The mildest GERD medications are antacids; these are generally the safest, cheapest, and have the least number of side effects of all GERD medications. You take antacids during episodes of reflux, and they work by neutralizing acid in the esophagus. A couple of examples of antacids are alumina/magnesia (Maalox) and calcium carbonate (Tums). Many different types and brands of antacids are available at your local pharmacy. Antacids are not very useful for preventing future GERD, though. Thus, antacids are generally recommended for rare or infrequent reflux.

For moderate and/or frequent GERD symptoms, it may be more beneficial and effective for you to take a medication regularly to prevent symptoms before they occur. Two other classes of medications treat GERD by decreasing or blocking stomach acid production. These are called H2 blockers and proton pump inhibitors. These classes of drugs represent the second and third tiers of GERD therapy, respectively. Generally speaking, they work on the premise of no acid, then no acid reflux. Side effects, cost, and strength of these drugs increase with each higher tier.

Most of these medications are available in some form over the counter; however, some may require a prescription. Usually, over-the-counter drugs are not covered by insurance prescription plans, so you might think there may be a financial benefit in obtaining a prescription from your doctor for GERD medication. However, insurance companies already understand this idea and respond by increasing co-payments for these agents, which gives you an incentive simply to pay for the over-the-counter drug.

Ideally, you should target GERD drug therapy to the degree of symptoms you have. Antacids may best treat periodic or rare reflux. If you have mild symptoms and know you are going out for Mexican or spicy food, taking an H2 blocker prior to the meal can be enough. If you get frequent, severe symptoms, a proton pump inhibitor is the drug of choice. Even if you do not get a prescription, you can always ask your doctor or local pharmacist for recommendations.

# PART FIVE

# Complications of Gastroesophageal Reflux Disease

What are the complications of GERD,
and are they serious?

What is regurgitation?

What is esophagitis?

*More...*

## 40. What are the complications of GERD, and are they serious?

Complications of GERD include those that occur in the esophagus and outside the esophagus (extra-esophageal complications) (see Figure 7). Esophageal complications include esophagitis (inflammation of the lining of the esophagus), **Barrett's esophagus**, narrowing or strictures, and, rarely, cancers. Extraesophageal complications can include sinus problems or infections, ringing in the ears, voice changes, dental problems, worsening of asthma, and recurrent pneumonia. Some of these complications are more like inconveniences; however, Barrett's esophagus, cancers, asthma, and pneumonias can be life-threatening. This is all the more reason to have GERD evaluated by a doctor. An expanded discussion of GERD complications follows.

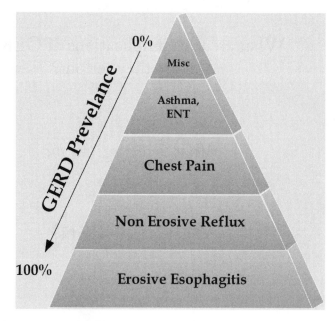

**Figure 7   GERD Pyramid.**

## 41. What is regurgitation?

Regurgitation is the sensation of material (food or liquid) coming up the esophagus (burping up material). This is usually worse just after eating when your stomach is full and there is more material to reflux up the esophagus. It is also worse at bedtime when you lie down. During the day, you have the benefit of gravity helping to keep things down in the stomach. When you lie down, the stomach and esophagus are level with each other, removing the effects of gravity, which facilitates material coming up and causing regurgitation.

*Regurgitation is the sensation of material (food or liquid) coming up the esophagus (burping up material).*

Regurgitation feels like liquid with an acidic or bitter taste coming up to the chest or mouth. Nighttime or nocturnal regurgitation can be very serious. During the day, when regurgitation occurs you are awake and can swallow it, protecting the windpipe and lungs. At night when you're asleep, this swallowing protection is not possible, and liquid can be inhaled into the lungs, causing aspiration that can lead to pneumonia.

Regurgitation can be prevented or minimized by eating smaller meals, not eating for at least 2 hours prior to going to bed, or elevating the head of the bed. Nighttime head elevation can be achieved by sleeping on a pillow that is wedge-shaped or by putting bricks or cinder blocks under the legs of the head of the bed.

Richard's comment:

*Regurgitation is very unpleasant, especially when it wakes you from a sound sleep. Not only is it uncomfortable, you know after it happens that it has to have serious health effects if not eliminated or substantially reduced. I have found that eating smaller dinners 3 to 4 hours before going to bed really helps the symptoms. I have also found that elevating my head while sleeping drastically reduces night-time acid reflux.*

## 42. What is esophagitis?

Esophagitis is inflammation of the lining of the esophagus that is diagnosed by a barium X-ray or endoscopy. Generally, it is not a diagnosis that can be made by a doctor in the office through a history or physical examination. The inflammation is usually caused by reflux of acid that burns, damaging the esophagus. However, medications can sometimes cause esophagitis, for example, aspirin or over-the-counter pain relievers, iron pills, potassium pills, some antibiotics, and certain drugs used to treat osteoporosis such as alendronate sodium. Rarely, infections of the lining of the esophagus such as yeast (*Candida*) or certain viruses can cause esophagitis. But again, generally most esophagitis is caused by acid reflux disease.

Symptoms of esophagitis are heartburn, occasionally chest pain, and/or difficulty swallowing. Treatment involves taking medication that suppresses acid production by the stomach, such as proton pump inhibitors like omeprazole (Prilosec) or a class of medications called **histamine-2 receptor antagonists** (or blockers) such as ranitidine (Zantac). Patients generally need 8 weeks of treatment to heal esophagitis, but most require some type of longer-term medication to maintain healing because there is a high risk of the inflammation returning after medication has been discontinued.

*Esophagitis is inflammation of the lining of the esophagus that is diagnosed by a barium X ray or endoscopy.*

In an endoscopic examination, a spectrum of inflammation can be seen and several grading scales are used to describe the severity of esophagitis. For example, the most commonly used scale is the **Los Angeles Esophagitis Grading Scale** (see Figure 8). This ranges from LA Grade A, which is mild redness at the bottom of the esophagus or mild esophagitis, to LA Grade D, which is severe inflammation with loss of some of the esophageal lining and severe ulceration. Despite the varying severity, the symptoms most patients experience are about the same. On rare occasions, patients with severe esophagitis can have nausea and vomiting. Very rarely, severe esophagitis can result in bleeding and anemia or low blood counts. Bleeding can manifest as vomiting frank blood or material that looks like coffee grounds, to passing blood in the stool

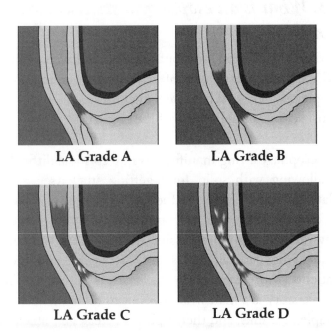

LA Grade A

LA Grade B

LA Grade C

LA Grade D

Figure 8    LA Classification.

that may look black and tarry. These symptoms warrant an urgent visit to the doctor or the closest emergency room because bleeding can be serious and requires immediate treatment.

Thankfully, most patients, even those with severe inflammation, heal readily when they take H2 blockers or PPI treatment. Sometimes severe esophagitis can heal but leave behind scarring and narrowing called strictures. Other times, when the esophagus heals, a new lining forms that is more resistant to acid damage; this condition is called Barrett's esophagus. Strictures and Barrett's esophagus present other problems that may require treatment and follow-up that are discussed later.

## 43. What is an esophageal stricture or ring?

Patients with and without chronic problems with GERD may be at risk of having a stricture or an esophageal ring. These are two different types of constrictions or narrowing of the esophagus.

An esophageal ring manifests as rare episodic difficulty swallowing with solid food getting stuck (see color plate 1). The sensation of food getting stuck can occur a couple times a year or may happen only once every few years. It is nonprogressive, meaning that over time swallowing generally does not get worse, and most patients with rings rarely have any symptoms. The classic story is a man who goes out to dinner and has a couple of drinks, and then a piece of steak gets stuck in his esophagus. This is called **steakhouse syndrome** and is caused by a structural narrowing at the bottom of the esophagus that interferes with swallowing for someone who has had a few drinks and is eating quickly or not chewing the food enough. Thus, a larger than normal swallowed piece of meat becomes stuck above the ring. This is an extremely uncomfortable situation: symptoms are mild chest pain, inability to swallow even saliva, and vomiting or regurgitation.

Sometimes with fluids the food passes, but frequently the person has to vomit the food to clear the blockage. If this does not work, then the person needs to go to the emergency room. Occasionally, medications can be taken to relax the esophagus so food can pass, but this usually does not work. Frequently, an emergent endoscopy test needs to be done to either remove the food or push it down into the stomach.

There is some debate in the medical literature as to whether esophageal rings are caused by chronic acid damage or whether people are born with them (congenital esophageal narrowing). Rings can easily be treated at the time of endoscopy. Rings generally occur at the bottom of the esophagus and at the top of a hiatal hernia where the lining of the esophagus and stomach meet. Local esophagitis or acid damage is not uncommon. Rings are very short and are composed of the superficial lining or mucosa of the esophagus. Esophageal rings are very common and do not always cause difficulty swallowing. If I endoscope a patient without a history of difficulty swallowing and I see a ring, I generally leave it alone. Rings are a benign process and do not get worse, cause esophagitis, or result in Barrett's esophagus or cancer.

*Rings are a benign process and do not get worse, cause esophagitis, or result in Barrett's esophagus or cancer.*

*Strictures are usually benign and result from chronic acid damage to the esophagus that causes the formation of scarring and contraction of the esophagus.*

An esophageal stricture is a different kind of esophageal narrowing (see color plate 2). Strictures generally do get worse with minor difficulty swallowing solids that may progress to extreme difficulty with solids or, rarely, solids and liquids. Strictures are usually benign and result from chronic acid damage to the esophagus that causes the formation of scarring and contraction of the esophagus. Rarely, a stricture can be caused by cancer (discussed later). Barium studies can diagnose a stricture but may not be able to tell whether it is benign or malignant, and frequently an endoscopy is needed to make the ultimate diagnosis.

Because strictures are caused by inflammation and chronic acid damage, they are longer and involve more of the esophagus than rings do. Strictures are scarring of not only the lining but also the wall of the esophagus. To allow healing they require more potent medication such as a PPI, which takes away the underlying cause of the stricture and allows the inflammation to resolve. Strictures are also treated at the time of endoscopy by stretching or dilating the esophagus. Some strictures can be very difficult to treat and can require repeat dilations.

*Pills may get stuck in the esophagus because they were taken dry or with inadequate water or because of a ring. When the pill sits there, it can burn, irritate, or ulcerate the esophagus, known as a pill ulcer.*

In addition to acid damage, some of the most difficult strictures can be caused by some medications (see table 2). Pills may get stuck in the esophagus because they were taken dry or with inadequate water or because of a ring. When the pill sits there, it can burn, irritate, or ulcerate the esophagus, known as a pill ulcer. Certain medications taken on a regular basis allow this process to happen repeatedly, resulting in scarring and a stricture.

**Table 2    Medications that Can Cause Direct Damage to the Esophagus**

| Medication (generic) | Medication (trade) | Uses |
| --- | --- | --- |
| Alendronate | Fosomax | Osteoporosis Medication |
| Aspirin | | Anti-inflammatory |
| Azithromycin | Zithromax | Antibiotic |
| Clarithromycin | Biaxin | Antibiotic |
| Erythromycin | E-mycin | Antibiotic |
| Ibuprofen | Advil, Motrin | Anti-inflammatory |
| Iron | | Mineral supplementation |
| Naproxen | Aleve, Naprosyn | Anti-inflammatory |
| Potassium | K-Dur | Mineral supplementation |
| Quinidine | Duraquin | Heart rate medication |
| Risedronate | Actonel | Osteoporosis medication |
| Tertracycline | Sumycin | Antibiotic |
| Vitamin C | | Vitamins |

## 44. What is an esophageal dilation?

**Esophageal dilation** is the technique of stretching the esophagus and is used to treat difficulty swallowing caused by strictures or rings. Most patients with GERD do not need dilation. It is done at the time of endoscopy while patients are sedated. Several different kinds of **dilators** and different tools are used for different jobs. Your doctor will choose the appropriate dilator based on the location of the narrowing, its length, how tight it is, and experience. We discuss only two kinds of dilators here.

The most commonly use dilator, which has been around for decades and the easiest to use is called a **Maloney dilator**. It is a long metal-weighted solid plastic tube with a tapered end and is reusable after sterilization. The Maloney dilator comes in various sizes to allow dilation of different kinds of narrowing of the esophagus. Usually, after the esophagus is examined with the **endoscope** a dilator is passed. This means that a very large hose-like object is swallowed to stretch the stricture. Sometimes multiple dilators need to be passed to ensure that the stricture or ring is adequately dilated. This dilator causes a controlled tear in the esophageal stricture. Although this sounds a like a medieval process, most patients do not remember it, it is not that uncomfortable, and is safe and effective in experienced hands.

Another type of dilator is a balloon dilator. This is literally a balloon on the end of a long thin tube that goes down the endoscope. Once the scope is positioned in the esophagus above the stricture, the balloon is advanced out of the scope and inflated, usually with water. There are different-sized balloons, and even single balloons can be inflated to different sizes based on need and how much pressure is injected into the balloon. The end result is the same as that of the Maloney dilator, a controlled tear in the stricture or ring is created.

Esophageal dilation is a very common procedure and is very safe. The risks are bleeding and perforation, or tearing a hole through the wall of the esophagus. Rarely—about 1 in 1,000 patients—can this happen. If

**Maloney dilator**

a tool used at the time of endoscopy to dilate or stretch out narrowing or strictures in the esophagus to improve swallowing.

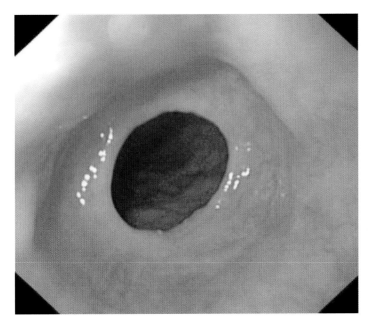

**Color Plate 1    Esophageal Ring**

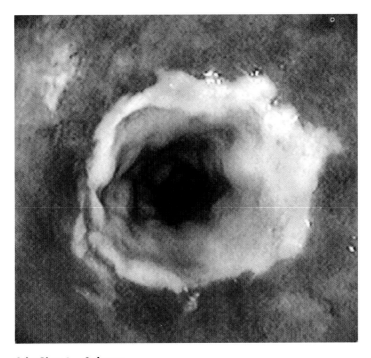

**Color Plate 2    Stricture**

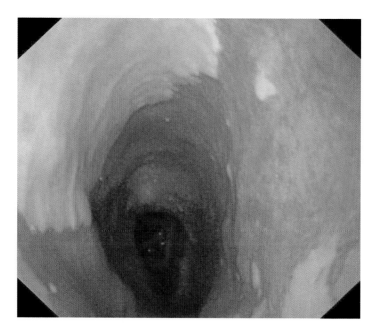

**Color Plate 3    Barrett's Esophagus**

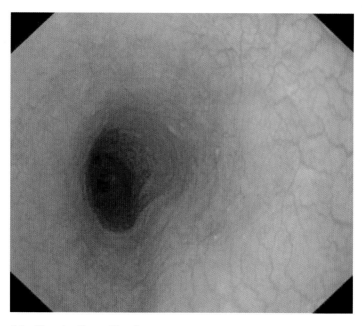

**Color Plate 4    Normal Esophagus**

this does occur, patients are hospitalized and generally undergo barium tests or a CAT scan to confirm the diagnosis. A surgeon sees the patient because surgery could be needed to repair the defect in the esophagus. Esophageal perforation is thankfully rare but is serious when it does occur, and a quick diagnosis is required. Esophageal bleeding after dilation is rare and could require hospitalization or a blood transfusion.

## 45. What is Barrett's esophagus?

Acid damage to the esophagus causes inflammation of the esophageal mucosa. This chronic inflammation can lead to a change in the mucosa to a different type that is more acid resistant. Barrett's, which can lead to cancer, is diagnosed during an endoscopy. This change can be diagnosed when an esophageal **biopsy** is examined under the microscope. (A **barium study** cannot make the diagnosis because a biopsy is required.) This abnormal acid-resistant lining is called **Barrett's esophagus** (see color plate 3). Barrett's esophagus is a concern because it predisposes you to esophageal cancer. A finding of Barrett's requires periodic follow-up with endoscopy and biopsy to determine whether any precancerous or cancerous changes have developed. These periodic tests can help diagnose esophageal cancer at an early stage or even possibly prevent it.

*Barrett's esophagus is a concern because it predisposes you to esophageal cancer.*

Most people with Barrett's esophagus have chronic heartburn or GERD symptoms. In fact, because Barrett's is more acid resistant, many patients report that their heartburn was worse when they were younger but is better now.

Many studies have examined the prevalence (how frequently it occurs) of Barrett's esophagus. An autopsy

*If you have chronic or long-standing heartburn symptoms and you are a white or Hispanic male between the ages of 40 and 60 years, you should see your doctor about an endoscopy test.*

study by Cameron and associates published in *Gastroenterology* in 1999 demonstrated a rate of 376 cases per 100,000 people. Barrett's is usually not found in young children and is thought to be an acquired condition. It is found predominantly in males that are middle-aged and is more common in Caucasians and Hispanics. Patients with chronic GERD undergoing endoscopy have been studied, and about 10–15% have Barrett's esophagus. About 40–50% of endoscoped patients have normal exams and the rest (about 40%) have esophagitis. Thus, if you have chronic or long-standing heartburn symptoms and you are a white or Hispanic male between the ages of 40 and 60 years, you should see your doctor about an endoscopy test.

Biopsies taken at endoscopy can reveal several different conditions that can resemble Barrett's, and this can be confusing even to some doctors. The biopsies are sent to a specialized doctor called a **pathologist**. These doctors spend years training to study various tissues under the microscope. The pathologist looks for very specific changes in the lining of the esophagus called **specialized intestinal metaplasia**. The lining of the esophagus changes to lining similar to that found in the small intestines; this is abnormal in the esophagus. The key to the diagnosis is the presence of special cells called **goblet cells**. These cells normally occur in the small intestine and other organs and produce mucus. So, the idea is that the biopsy must show goblet cells; if there are no goblet cells, there is no Barrett's.

## 46. Will I get cancer from having Barrett's esophagus?

As mentioned, Barrett's is an abnormal lining of the esophagus made of cells that are usually found elsewhere in the gut and it can predispose you to esophageal cancer. In the medical literature, many studies examine the association between cancer risk and Barrett's esophagus. Studies demonstrate an annual risk of getting cancer at 0.2–2% or on average about 0.5% per year. Another way to look at this is if 200 people have Barrett's esophagus, one person will get cancer each year. It is felt that the risk of getting esophageal cancer if you have Barrett's is increased thirtyfold over people who do not have Barrett's. Although when most people hear this they think they are going to die from cancer; fortunately uncommon things happen uncommonly.

*Studies demonstrate an annual risk of getting cancer at 0.2–2% or on average about 0.5% per year.*

Annually in the United States approximately 8,000 people get the cancer associated with Barrett's esophagus called **adenocarcinoma**. Another kind of esophageal cancer is called **squamous cell carcinoma**. These cancers generally behave the same and unfortunately commonly can cause death. Under the microscope, they are different and can be treated differently. The risk factors for these two cancers are different as well. Squamous cell cancers are believed to be caused more by smoking and excessive alcohol use.

Now the good news: all cancer statistics have to be put in perspective. Esophageal cancer is rare even if you have Barrett's esophagus. The American Cancer Society Web site reports that in 2004, 230,000 men had prostate cancer, 216,000 women had breast cancer, 174,000 people had lung cancer, and 150,000 people had colon cancer. Esophageal cancer does not even rank in the top eight types of cancer in the United States annually. When you look at it from a more global perspective, of the more than 1,350,000 new

*Doctors routinely screen for cancer, prostate checks, breast exams and pap smears, and colon cancer screening. For a patient with Barrett's esophagus, periodic endoscopy and biopsies are added to the cancer screening routine, and the condition really is just another chronic medical problem.*

cancer diagnoses in 2004, only 14,000 cases were esophageal cancer, and half of those were associated with Barrett's esophagus. Or consider it this way: of all the cancers in the United States in 2004, half of 1% (1 in 200 cancers) were associated with Barrett's. When I give patients the diagnosis of Barrett's esophagus, I tell them to relax. Even with Barrett's, the risk of getting other cancers completely unrelated to the esophagus is much higher than is the risk of getting a cancer associated with Barrett's. Doctors routinely screen for cancer, including prostate checks for men, mammograms, breast exams and pap smears for women, and colon cancer screening for those age 50 and older. For a patient with Barrett's esophagus, periodic endoscopy and biopsies are added to the cancer screening routine, and the condition really is just another chronic medical problem.

The major issue with esophageal cancer is that generally it is a serious cancer that is usually found late and at an advanced stage. In 2004, 14,250 esophageal cancers were diagnosed; about half were adenocarcinoma. There were 13,300 deaths from esophageal cancer that year. More than 90% of people diagnosed with esophageal cancer die of it. (These data are available on the American Cancer Society Web site if you want more information.)

Barrett's increases cancer risk because the repeated inflammation and injury with periodic healing damages the **DNA** of the abnormal esophageal lining. The DNA is the code within cells that regulates growth and cell division. When the DNA is damaged, it can result in cells with abnormal growth patterns that do not reproduce normally and that can evolve into cancer.

You may be able to decrease your cancer risk by avoiding smoking, limiting alcohol use, maintaining a healthy weight, eating a balanced diet that includes fruits and vegetables, taking heartburn medication, and getting periodic endoscopy if Barrett's has developed. If you have questions, a lot of information is available, so ask your doctor.

## 47. What can be done to make Barrett's esophagus better or make it go away?

The short answer is nothing. There is some debate in the literature whether Barrett's will regress, shrink, or go away with aggressive antacid treatment or with surgery for GERD. But the information is mixed; some doctors feel that regular use of antacid drugs such as proton pump inhibitors (for example, omeprazole) may decrease the amount of Barrett's lining the esophagus. It has been clearly demonstrated that the more of the esophagus lined by Barrett's, the greater the cancer risk.

*It has been clearly demonstrated that the more of the esophagus lined by Barrett's, the greater the cancer risk.*

My recommendation to patients is that surgery for GERD does not improve Barrett's once it has developed. Most patients with Barrett's have heartburn; if I make the diagnosis of Barrett's, I tend to treat them with daily or twice daily doses of proton pump inhibitors. There really is no downside, and such treatment may limit progression of Barrett's, but the data in the literature to support this are not conclusive. The disadvantages of this approach are drug cost and the requirement of taking regular medication. This class of medications is safe to take long term and has few side effects.

Endoscopic studies that look at different ways to treat Barrett's are under way. There are techniques using various tools to cauterize, burn off, or ablate Barrett's, but as of yet it is unclear whether these work or reduce cancer risk.

## 48. If I have Barrett's esophagus, does it need to be followed?

Yes, it does need to be followed with periodic endoscopy and biopsy. Barrett's can degenerate into cancer in stages. Within Barrett's when precancerous changes can be seen, this is called **dysplasia** and is further broken down into low-grade and **high-grade dysplasia**. This spectrum from Barrett's to low-grade to high-grade dysplasia and then cancer can be diagnosed on biopsy. Dysplasia represents progressive damage to the DNA within cells, which become more irregular and abnormal. If patients have "normal" Barrett's, then the cancer risk is low, but this increases with the presence of dysplasia.

According to the American College of Gastroenterology, the following maintenance schedule for endoscopy is recommended. All patients should be on antacid medications prior to endoscopy to eliminate any inflammation of the esophagus, which might cloud the diagnosis. Patients diagnosed with Barrett's on endoscopy should have another endoscopy one year later to ensure no changes have developed. Then they should have endoscopy and biopsies every 3 years. If low-grade or mild dysplasia is found, then yearly endoscopy and biopsy should be done. If high-grade dysplasia is found, this can be a marker of cancer and the situation becomes very complicated. The short

*Patients diagnosed with Barrett's on endoscopy should have another endoscopy one year later to ensure no changes have developed. Then they should have endoscopy and biopsies every 3 years.*

answer is surgery to remove the esophagus may be needed but for the sake of discussion other options may be available.

The benefit of this recommended surveillance endoscopy for Barrett's is that dysplasia can be diagnosed and followed more closely before cancer develops. If cancer does occur, it can be detected long before it would have caused any symptoms. Therefore, if it is diagnosed at an earlier stage, it becomes more treatable or curable.

## 49. What are the "alarm" or concerning symptoms that might suggest esophageal cancer?

Unfortunately, when esophageal cancer causes symptoms, the cancer is usually too advanced for treatment or cure and options may be limited (see Table 3). This is demonstrated by the fact that more than 90% of

*Unfortunately, when esophageal cancer causes symptoms, the cancer is usually too advanced for treatment or cure and options may be limited.*

**Table 3    GERD Alarm Signs Suggesting Workup**

| Alarm Signs |
| --- |
| Progressive difficulty swallowing |
| Black-to-bloody bowel movements |
| Vomiting blood |
| Weight loss |
| Choking sensation |
| Chest pain |

those diagnosed with esophageal cancer die of their disease. Hopefully, by doing endoscopy on people with chronic heartburn and diagnosing Barrett's esophagus, this mortality rate can be improved by identifying precancer or cancerous changes earlier.

The symptoms of esophageal cancer are difficulty swallowing solids with the sensation of food getting stuck. This is progressive, meaning that it starts with occasional difficulty that then gets worse until there is a problem swallowing solids, liquids, or even saliva. You may feel achy or have vague chest pain or discomfort. Most, if not all patients, with symptomatic esophageal cancer lose weight because the cancer produces substances that suppress the appetite. Some patients have an unexplained low level of blood or anemia.

No blood tests can diagnose esophageal cancer. It cannot be diagnosed in a doctor's office by a physical examination. Esophageal cancer is usually diagnosed by a barium study that demonstrates an abnormality in the esophagus or by endoscopy.

## 50. How can I decrease my risk of getting cancer of the esophagus?

*Overall, you can do some easy things to decrease cancer risk, esophageal or otherwise.*

Overall, you can do some easy things to decrease cancer risk, esophageal or otherwise. Avoid smoking or chewing tobacco and limit your alcohol use. Two-thirds of all Americans are overweight, which is associated with an increased risk of certain cancers. Thus, trying to maintain an ideal weight may reduce cancer risk and will certainly decrease your risk of high blood pressure, heart disease, stroke, abnormal cholesterol, and diabetes. Eat fresh fruits and vegetables and avoid foods that contain preservatives. Fresh foods contain chemicals such as vitamins, minerals, and antioxidants that have a protective benefit. Regular exercise helps to maintain a healthy weight and decreases risk. Some vitamin supplements, such as calcium, folic acid, and antioxidants like selenium have demonstrated decreased cancer risks.

Specifically for esophageal cancer, tobacco and alcohol are the major factors you can modify to decrease the chances of developing cancer. For patients with chronic GERD, endoscopy, as previously mentioned, can help diagnose cancer at an earlier stage or may help to diagnose Barrett's esophagus. Some studies show that aspirin or a class of drugs called NSAIDs (most over-the-counter pain relievers, except acetaminophen [Tylenol]) can decrease the risk of developing cancer in patients with Barrett's esophagus.

## 51. What is aspiration?

Reflux is the movement of fluid and/or food from the stomach up into the esophagus. In the back of throat are the openings to the esophagus and the airway to the lungs called the trachea. When you breathe, this valve opens, allowing air into the trachea and lungs (see Figure 12). When you eat, the epiglottis in the back of the throat closes so that food material does not pass into the trachea (see Figure 13). Sometimes when you eat, liquids particularly might "go down the wrong pipe," and you start coughing. This process of liquid entering the trachea is called aspiration; coughing is the body's

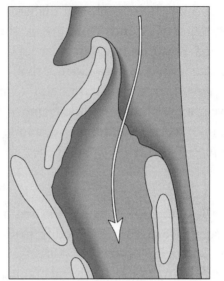

Trachea    Esophagus

**Figure 12    Airway.**

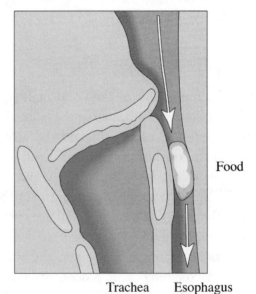

Food

Trachea    Esophagus

**Figure 13    Swallowing Food.**

way of clearing material from the trachea. The trachea and esophagus lie right next to each other. If reflux happens occasionally, it can travel all the way up the esophagus and enter the trachea, and that is also called aspiration.

The risk of aspiration is particularly increased at night when you are lying down and do not have the benefit of gravity helping to keep material in the stomach. Nighttime aspiration is common in those with reflux. The classic symptom is waking from sleep coughing, choking, wheezing, or tasting bitter material in your mouth. Most of the time this is scary and a nuisance, but if the liquid travels down to the lungs, you can have more serious problems, such as aspiration pneumonia. Aspiration pneumonia is a type of pneumonia (an infection of the lungs) caused by irritating acidic material entering and damaging the lungs. Sometimes you may need to take antibiotics to treat aspiration pneumonia; occasionally the condition can be very serious and require hospitalization. Chronic aspiration can also damage the trachea and lungs and make chronic lung disease or asthma worse.

There are ways to minimize the risk of nighttime reflux and aspiration. Avoid food for 2 hours prior to bed to allow the stomach to empty and to eliminate material to aspirate. Because there is no food or less food in the stomach, the pressure in the stomach is lower and the force promoting reflux is diminished. Elevating the head of the bed and sleeping on an incline can help use gravity to keep material down in the stomach. Special wedge-shaped pillows keep the head and chest above the level of the stomach. Antacid medications that will help with nighttime heartburn

*There are ways to minimize the risk of nighttime reflux and aspiration. Avoid food for 2 hours prior to bed to allow the stomach to empty and to eliminate material to aspirate.*

and aspiration can be taken at bedtime. Avoid certain foods and drinks —chocolate, caffeine from coffee or tea, and alcohol—at night or just before you sleep, because these relax the lower esophageal sphincter (the muscular valve at the bottom of the esophagus).

## 52. What is laryngopharyngeal reflux?

*Laryngopharyngeal reflux (LPR)* is a term used by doctors to describe reflux that damages the larynx, which is the voice box and entrance to the trachea. The **pharynx** is the part of the throat that becomes the esophagus. If you experience changes in your voice, you might see an ear, nose, and throat doctor. To evaluate voice problems, a small camera is passed up the nose and down into the larynx (the voice box) to examine the area. LPR is a frequent cause of damage to the voice box caused by reflux of stomach acid. Usually this is treated with antacid medication. If severe, LPR can result in narrowing of the trachea, irritation of the voice box, the development of growths or polyps, and in rare cases, cancer of the larynx.

*Reflux and LPR are risk factors for laryngeal cancer in non-smokers.*

Smoking is the major cause of cancer of the larynx; however, this type of cancer can occur in nonsmokers. Reflux and LPR are risk factors for laryngeal cancer in nonsmokers.

## 53. Is there a relationship between GERD and asthma or chronic lung disease?

Fifteen million Americans have asthma, and it is estimated that about 30–90% of asthmatics have reflux. Asthma is a lung disease characterized by muscle spasms in the airways of the lungs. When these muscles go into spasm and contract, it limits the ability of air to move in or out of the lungs and causes wheezing, shortness of breath, or coughing. This is treated usually with inhaled medications that relax the airways. Many factors can start an asthma attack, such as pollen and other allergens such as animal hair, cold air, noxious fumes, and stomach acid. Sometimes a chest cold caused by an infection can start or worsen asthma symptoms.

Some people with asthma have symptoms of GERD, but many do not. A study of 199 asthmatics who had **pH** studies (see Question 69) conducted by Harding, Guzzon, and Richter, and published in *Chest* in 1999, showed that 72% had abnormal amounts of acid in the esophagus. Reflux makes asthma worse when aspirated stomach acid enters the lungs and burns the airways, causing these muscles to go into spasm. A large portion of the patients studied reported no reflux symptoms. So, asthmatics may have a problem with silent reflux and not even know it.

*Reflux makes asthma worse when aspirated stomach acid enters the lungs and burns the airways, causing these muscles to go into spasm.*

Other studies of patients with asthma have shown improvement of asthma symptoms and decreased need for asthma medications for those treated with antacid medications. Because of this, many lung doctors recommend a 3-month trial of antacid medication for asthma patients with obvious GERD. Antacid medications might also be considered for those with poorly controlled asthma that requires multiple medications.

## 54. Is there a relationship between GERD and a chronic cough?

Chronic coughing is defined as the presence of a cough for more than 3 weeks and is one of the most common reasons for which people seek medical attention. A cough is a vigorous contraction or shortening of the muscles for breathing that results in a high-pressure movement of air out of the lungs. The purpose of a cough is to clear mucus, particles, or irritants from the lungs or airways. Nerves in the throat and airways can sense mucus and irritants such as noxious fumes, allergens such as pollen, or stomach acid. When these nerves are stimulated a message is sent to the brain and a cough is stimulated.

There are several causes of chronic coughing. Some people with asthma do not have the usual symptoms of shortness of breath or wheezing and may only have coughing. Postnasal drip with mucus dripping down the throat can cause a chronic cough. Obviously, infections such as bronchitis or pneumonia can cause coughing. GERD or laryngopharyngeal reflux (see Question 52) can cause a chronic cough. Acid, which is a potent irritant, refluxes up the esophagus and into the larynx (the voice box) and the airways. This stimulates the nerves that line these structures and causes a cough in an attempt by the body to clear the offending irritant. It is felt that GERD is probably responsible for 30–40% of chronic coughing. Of those with GERD-related cough, about two-thirds have heartburn symptoms but a third do not.

*GERD with or without symptoms plays a major role in many lung diseases such as asthma, chronic cough, aspiration, pneumonia, and LPR.*

GERD with or without symptoms plays a major role in many lung diseases such as asthma, chronic cough, aspiration, pneumonia, and LPR. It may be reasonable for you to try taking antacid medication for a few months to see if these conditions can be improved, even in the absence of obvious GERD symptoms.

Alternatively, if GERD is suspected, testing can be done. A barium study (see Question 61) may show reflux of barium up into the airways or lungs. A **pH study**, which measures the presence of acid in the esophagus, can also be helpful in diagnosing GERD in patients with chronic cough or lung symptoms.

## 55. Does GERD play a role in chronic chest pain?

There are many causes of chest pain because many structures "live" in the chest. The chest wall, the muscles, ribs, and cartilage can cause pain. Chest pain may be related to the heart or lungs or the esophagus. The types and character of the discomfort related to these organs are generally different but can be quite similar in some individuals. Sometimes it can be very difficult to tell whether the chest pain a patient is experiencing is a heart attack or just heartburn. Because of this *have a doctor immediately evaluate any chest pain or discomfort.* Heart attacks can be treated, and patients absolutely need to be evaluated for the presence of impaired blood flow to the heart. This can be a matter of life and death. That said, if you have chest pain or discomfort, have been evaluated by a doctor, and have had heart problems tested for and ruled out, then GERD may be the issue. This is called noncardiac ("not heart") chest pain.

Symptoms of esophageal chest pain are pain after a meal, pain after drinking very cold liquids, pain associated with difficulty swallowing, or pain improved with antacid medications. If this is the case, a trial of medication such as a high-dose proton pump inhibitor

*Sometimes it can be very difficult to tell whether the chest pain a patient is experiencing is a heart attack or just heartburn. Because of this have a doctor immediately evaluate any chest pain or discomfort.*

should be tried, for example, omeprazole 20 milligrams twice a day. If there is improvement of symptoms, this suggests that there may be an esophageal cause for the chest pain.

Alternatively, if there is no change or minimal improvement, other tests can be done. Acid or pH testing is abnormal in approximately 60% of those with noncardiac chest pain, suggesting GERD as a cause of the pain. Esophageal motility testing (see Question 68) may be helpful. This test can diagnose muscle spasms in the esophagus, which feel like severe, crushing chest pain that can last for minutes and feel like a heart attack. Different substances can be dripped into the esophagus during the testing to see whether the chest pain symptoms can be provoked or caused. An example, called a **Bernstein test,** is when acid (like stomach acid) is infused into the esophagus during a motility test. This allows for pressure measurement in the esophagus to see if muscle spasms occur and the patient can subjectively tell the tester whether he or she is having chest pain during the acid challenge.

As mentioned, treatment for noncardiac chest pain first is a high-dose proton pump inhibitor (PPI) antacid. If this fails, you can try another PPI or other drugs such as muscle relaxers or even some antidepressant medications.

Richard's comment:

*I do not have chronic chest pain or many of the other serious side effects of acid reflux. Having become familiar with these terrible symptoms (i.e., chronic coughing, difficulty swallowing food, Barrett's esophagus, chronic heartburn, larynx problems), I am determined to control my acid reflux with smart lifestyle changes.*

## 56. Is there a relationship between GERD and cancers of the head and neck?

Cancer of the head and neck is the fifth most common cancer in the United States. The head and neck includes the mouth, tongue, nose, nasopharynx, sinuses, pharynx, tonsils, and larynx. The most common cancer site in the head and neck is the larynx or voice box. This accounts for about a quarter of all head and neck cancers. The greatest risk factor for head and neck cancer is smoking; however, cancer of the larynx increasingly is being reported in patients who were lifetime nonsmokers.

As previously discussed, reflux can affect the larynx (see Question 52). Long-standing acid damage to the larynx causes inflammation of the cells lining the larynx. Repeated damage and healing causes these cells to die off and reproduce themselves at a faster rate than normal. Because of this faster turnover of cells, there is a greater risk of damage to the DNA (the genetic code within the cells), which allows cells to become more and more abnormal as they reproduce and ultimately results in cancer. Signs and symptoms of laryngeal cancer are a long-standing sore throat or voice changes such as hoarseness. A doctor specializing in diseases of the ears, nose, and throat, an ENT doctor, usually makes the diagnosis.

# PART SIX

# *Doctor's Evaluation*

When should I see my doctor about my GERD symptoms?

What kind of doctor treats GERD?

What symptoms should prompt a doctor's evaluation?

*More...*

## 57. When should I see my doctor about my GERD symptoms?

You should see your doctor about GERD or heartburn before waiting too long. A burning chest discomfort may be GERD or it could be something else such as a heart problem. Angina or heart pain can be difficult to differentiate from GERD. If you are not sure or have any questions, this should prompt a visit to your doctor, especially if the discomfort is associated with shortness of breath, dizziness, sweating, and/or arm or jaw pain or if the chest discomfort is associated with exercise. People with risk factors associated with heart disease such as a family history of heart attacks, smokers, those with high blood pressure, and those with high cholesterol are at increased risk for heart disease, and any chest pain warrants a doctor visit.

*Angina or heart pain can be difficult to differentiate from GERD. If you are not sure or have any questions, this should prompt a visit to your doctor*

Assuming the GERD is really just heartburn, any of the following requires a visit to your doctor:

- If you have had problems with GERD for more than a few months and are regularly taking over-the-counter medications. You may want to see your doctor because there may be better or more appropriate medications.
- If you experience GERD symptoms three times or more per week. This frequency may increase GERD complications.
- If you have *any* difficulty swallowing, with food or liquids getting stuck.
- If you wake at night coughing or choking or experience increased symptoms of asthma. This may be a manifestation of GERD.

- If you experience recurrent sinus infections, unexplained changes in voice such as hoarseness, or ringing in the ears (also called tinnitus). This may be atypical manifestations of GERD.

Any one of these symptoms can be treated and should be evaluated by a doctor because further testing or medication may be in order.

## 58. What kind of doctor treats GERD?

Your primary care doctor should do the initial evaluation of GERD. This kind of doctor is usually an internist or doctor who does general internal medicine and only treats adults. Other primary care doctors might be family practitioners who treat both adults and children. Your doctor may treat you with medication for GERD and/or order tests.

If you are on medication that is not working or have any of the symptoms from the preceding question, your doctor may refer you to a **gastroenterologist**. Gastroenterologists are doctors who have trained in adult internal medicine and have done several years of additional training in diseases of the digestive tract, liver, and pancreas. They generally see patients in the office and do various procedures. These procedures are usually upper endoscopy and colonoscopy. Upper endoscopy involves passing instruments down through the mouth to examine the esophagus, stomach, and duodenum and can be used to evaluate GERD. A colonoscopy is a screening test for colon cancer.

Depending on where you live and the availability of specialist doctors, surgeons or family practitioners may perform procedures. You may be referred to one of these doctors for an upper endoscopy test for evaluation of your GERD.

## 59. What symptoms should prompt a doctor's evaluation?

Frequent GERD, occurring three or more times a week or longstanding symptoms of more than 6 months may be a sign of damage to the esophagus. Acid damage of the esophagus called esophagitis is present in about half of patients who have an endoscopy test. About 5–10% may have Barrett's esophagus (see color plate 3). Barrett's esophagus is an inflammatory change in the lining of the esophagus that can predispose you to the development of esophageal cancer.

*Frequent GERD, occurring three or more times a week or longstanding symptoms of more than 6 months may be a sign of damage to the esophagus.*

If you have difficulty swallowing and experience the sensation of food getting stuck in your chest, you should see your doctor. Acid damage to the esophagus can cause scarring or narrowing of the esophagus called strictures or rings. Generally, symptoms may be caused by food, particularly solid food when it becomes stuck. These symptoms may be present for years and might occur infrequently. Occasionally, solids and liquids both may be difficult to swallow. Food can also get stuck and sometimes you may not be able to get the material all the way down to the stomach. You may need to vomit or regurgitate the retained material. Sometimes food can become completely stuck and a doctor may need to remove it in the emergency room or hospital.

Progressive difficulty swallowing solids that requires you to make changes in diet such as cutting food into smaller and smaller pieces, avoiding foods such as meats, and grinding up food may be signs of problems. Particularly if these symptoms are associated with weight loss and/or chest pain, it is important to seek medical attention. These symptoms may be a sign of esophageal cancer. Generally, when patients have cancer, one of the last symptoms to develop is difficulty swallowing. Unfortunately, this results in cancers being discovered at a late or advanced stage.

It can be very difficult to tell whether the symptom of difficulty swallowing is caused by a benign process like a stricture or ring that can be easily treated or by an esophageal cancer. Thus, it is very important that a doctor evaluate any swallowing problems so the cause can quickly be diagnosed and treated.

## 60. Should I just have a trial of medication for GERD?

If you experience GERD symptoms or heartburn rarely or infrequently, over-the-counter medication is a good place to start. Antacids may be helpful for more rarely experienced symptoms. For more frequent or severe symptoms, drugs called H2 blockers such as ranitidine, cimetidine (Tagamet), and famotidine (Pepcid) can be used. For more severe GERD, omeprazole (Prilosec-OTC) can be used. However, omeprazole is approved for use only for 14 days. All of these medications are over the counter (OTC) and do not require a doctor's prescription. Generally, for mild to moderate GERD symptoms, a trial of medication is reasonable.

If you have ongoing symptoms despite a trial of medication, then visit your doctor. Many different medications are available for treatment of GERD, both over the counter and by prescription. Generally speaking, the prescription drugs are stronger and work better for more severe symptoms. Also, some medications are effective only when taken appropriately. For example, the class of GERD drugs called proton pump inhibitors (PPIs) such as omeprazole need to be taken 30 to 45 minutes prior to eating to get maximum effect. So, if you have rare or infrequent heartburn and you take a PPI while having symptoms, it generally does not work because you have taken it the wrong way. A more effective medication to take during symptoms might be an OTC antacid. This is an example of why a doctor's visit can be helpful.

# PART SEVEN

# Testing for GERD

What is a barium study or upper GI series?

What is a pH study and why is it done?

Is an endoscopy painful, and does it carry risks?

*More...*

## 61. *What is a barium study or upper GI series?*

If you see a doctor, he or she may recommend evaluation of GERD symptoms or difficulty swallowing. A barium study is one of these tests. It goes by multiple names such as **upper GI series**, barium swallow, or barium esophagram. This is a simple and easy test that is usually done at a hospital in the X-ray or radiology department. It involves drinking a liquid material that may be chalky tasting that is closely followed by an X-ray examination. The entire exam usually takes less than 30 minutes. Normally, the esophagus and upper gastroesophageal tract cannot be seen well on X-ray. However, the barium liquid coats the lining of the esophagus, stomach, and small intestine, which allows careful examination. Sometimes the doctor or technician may ask you to take something called **fizzies**. This is a material that produces gas and helps to distend your stomach so it can be more carefully examined. Rarely, you may need an intravenous line (IV) to administer other medications, but generally an IV is used for examination of the small intestine, which is not an issue when evaluating for GERD.

A barium study is painless (unless you get an IV, which is only minimally painful). The amount of radiation is relatively small. When you are flying in an airplane, you are exposed to cosmic radiation; your radiation exposure during an upper GI exam is roughly equal to that of two round-trip flights from New York to Los Angeles. This is a small amount of radiation and should not be of concern.

A barium exam can be very helpful and give a lot of information. Inflammation of the esophagus can be detected. Ulcers, strictures, scarring, rings, and cancers can be found. It can also give your doctor direction if further testing is needed.

## 62. What is an endoscopy?

When patients have had frequent or long-standing GERD symptoms, they can develop inflammatory changes to the esophagus called Barrett's esophagus that can predispose them to esophageal cancer. The only way to make the diagnosis of Barrett's is to do an endoscopy test. Difficulty swallowing can be evaluated and treated at the time of endoscopy.

An endoscopy test is usually done at a hospital or an ambulatory **endoscopy center**, which is a freestanding facility not associated with a hospital. An endoscope is a long, thin instrument that includes a light and a video camera that can be guided into narrow and small organs. Air and water can be passed into the endoscope and sucked out, allowing for cleaning retained material or mucus. Tools can be passed down the endoscope for tissue sampling, treatment of bleeding, and dilation of the esophagus. Tiny **forceps** can be used to take biopsies or long, thin balloons can be passed through the scope to dilate strictures. Video or still pictures can be taken with most endoscopes.

Generally, a gastroenterologist performs endoscopy, but in some parts of the country general surgeons or other physicians perform them. The test evaluates the esophagus, stomach, and duodenum (the first part of the small intestine). During the exam, biopsies can be taken if needed.

If you are getting an endoscopy, you will be asked not to eat or drink anything after midnight the night before the test so your stomach will be empty. Your doctor may request you make minor changes in your medication; for example, you might hold off taking blood thinners such as clopidogrel (Plavix), warfarin (Coumadin), or aspirin for a few days prior to the examination. Also, diabetic patients must change their insulin dosing. *Do not make any medication changes on your own—ask your doctor.* Also, do not go to an endoscopy test alone. You will likely be sedated and given medication for relaxation or sleep and will not be able to drive after the test. Someone will need to drive you home.

*Do not make any medication changes on your own—ask your doctor.*

Overall, from arrival to leaving is about 2 hours. A nurse or doctor will interview you, asking about your medical history, medications that you are taking, symptoms, and drug allergies. Your mouth, heart, lungs, and abdomen will be examined. An IV is placed so that the sedative medication can be given. Then, you will be brought into the procedure room. Monitors for oxygen levels, heart rhythm and rate, and blood pressure will be placed on your arms and chest. You will get supplemental oxygen because some people do not breathe as well while sedated. All of this occurs prior to starting the actual endoscopy test.

Once all of the preparation is complete, a nurse or anesthesiologist will administer the sedative. Patients may sleep through the exam and may not remember it, or they may be sleepy—it depends on the doctor and medications used for sedation. The mouth is usually sprayed or you will gargle with a topical anesthetic to numb the throat so the instrument can be easily passed. The topical anesthetic also helps to prevent you from gagging and is generally very effective even with patients who gag easily. Once sedated, an endoscope is passed into your mouth, down the esophagus, into the stomach and duodenum. The actual test takes only about 10 to 15 minutes. Endoscopy allows for direct visualization of the lining of the esophagus, and little pieces of tissue can painlessly be removed (biopsied) for analysis. If there is narrowing of the esophagus, it can be treated or dilated at this time.

After the exam patients are brought to a recovery room and will sleep off the sedative, which may take about 30 to 60 minutes. This is really the only "recovery" from the exam you need because no cuts or incisions are made and no pain results from the test. Most doctors recommend that you not drive, work, exercise, consume alcohol, or make important decisions the day of the exam because it takes about 24 hours for the medication to completely clear from your system. It is important that you avoid alcohol for 24 hours because it can interact with the medication that remains in your system.

## 63. Is an endoscopy painful, and does it carry risks?

Endoscopy is a safe and routine procedure. The major risks involve the anesthesia. On rare occasions, patients can have allergic reactions to the medications. The anesthetic risks are generally cardiac and pulmonary, or heart- and lung-related. Examples are irregular heart rates or, very rarely, heart attacks. These complications may occur in patients with a history of heart disease or lung disease. The major risk for the actual endoscopy is bleeding or perforation. A perforation is a tear in the lining of the esophagus or stomach. On rare occasions, this can require a hospital stay,

*Endoscopy is a safe and routine procedure.*

blood transfusion, or surgery to fix the tear. All of these risks or complications are exceedingly rare: less than 1 in 1000 procedures.

Overall, an endoscopy is not painful—no cutting or incisions are made. The placement of an IV is slightly uncomfortable but quick. Sometimes the initial passage of the scope through the throat into the esophagus is a little uncomfortable because it is an unusual feeling to swallow the endoscope. I have had an endoscopy, and I do not remember a thing about it and did not find it to be an unpleasant experience (DLB).

The most common issue patients experience is a sore throat that lasts for a couple days after the procedure. This is because the scope travels through the back of the throat and can cause some irritation. The other issue may be some dizziness or nausea after the endoscopy. This is related to the sedative medication because side effects can include some nausea. This is easily treated and usually is short-lived.

One issue patients often ask about is the risk of infection or catching something from the exam. This is very rare because endoscopes are cleaned carefully with sterilizing solutions pumped through the instrument between examinations. Yes, endoscopes are reused many times, but their cleaning is standardized and regulated by federal agencies that license hospitals and freestanding endoscopy units or surgical centers.

Finally, before your endoscopy, the nurse or preferably the doctor will go over the risks and benefits of the examination with you. This is an opportunity to discuss issues and ask questions. You will then sign a form called an **informed consent**. The informed consent states the risks of the exam, and by signing you are acknowledging that you understand the risks and agree to go ahead with the procedure.

Richard's comment:

*I have had two endoscopies over the last 5 years. On both occasions, the procedure was uneventful and, in fact, I do not remember anything from the procedure itself. Mine were done by a gastroenterologist, and I felt very comfortable with the information presented to me and the care I received from the nursing staff. There is no reason I would not have another endoscopy if my doctor felt it necessary.*

## 64. Do I need a biopsy of the esophagus, and does it hurt?

It is fairly common to do biopsies during an endoscopy. A small biopsy forceps is passed down the endoscope and a tiny pinch of tissue is removed. This is sent to a pathologist, who examines the tissue under a microscope. This can be extremely helpful for the evaluation of patients with GERD. A normal-appearing esophagus on endoscopy can have microscopic clues to the presence of reflux disease. Abnormal areas can be biopsied to check for cancer.

As previously mentioned, chronic reflux can put you at risk for a precancerous condition called Barrett's esophagus. This is an irreversible change in the lining of the esophagus resulting from chronic acid damage. Barrett's esophagus cannot be diagnosed with a barium or upper GI study. An endoscopy can only suggest whether Barrett's esophagus may or may not be present. In fact, the only way to make the definitive diagnosis is by taking a biopsy and looking for certain changes under the microscope. So, for the diagnosis of Barrett's a biopsy is mandatory.

Biopsies of the esophagus (or for that matter anywhere in the gut) do not hurt. The nerves of the gut do not feel cutting or burning. But they do feel stretching, pulling, and distention from the scope or air that is used during the procedure.

## 65. Should I be checked for H. pylori at the endoscopy?

**Helicobacter pylori (H. pylori)**

a bacterium that lives in the stomach and can cause stomach ulcers. It is diagnosed usually by biopsy of the stomach and treated with 10 to 14 days of antibiotics and antacid medication. The role of *H. pylori* in GERD is unclear.

As discussed earlier, an endoscopic biopsy is a benign and painless procedure. *Helicobacter pylori (H. pylori)* is the bacterium that causes ulcers and predisposes you to the development of stomach cancer. Thus, finding and treating *H. pylori* is desirable. Generally, biopsies are done for *H. pylori* in patients who have ulcers or a history of prior ulcers because they may have a chronic *H. pylori* infection. Those with stomach irritation on endoscopy, a family history of stomach cancer, or dyspepsia should be evaluated for *H. pylori*. Dyspepsia is a combination of symptoms that resemble an ulcer in the absence of an ulcer and is characterized by upper abdominal discomfort such as burning or gnawing that is improved with antacid medication. Some doctors check all patients for *H. pylori* when they do an endoscopy. When it is found, *H. pylori* should be treated, which involves about 2 weeks of medication. *H. pylori* therapy usually includes three drugs: an antacid and two antibiotics.

## 66. What does an endoscopy show when patients have GERD?

Patients with chronic GERD symptoms undergoing endoscopy have been studied by Winters and colleagues. In a report published in *Gastroenterology* in 1987, the authors found that of approximately 100 patients with longstanding or chronic GERD who had an upper endoscopy, 42% were normal, 45% demonstrated erosive esophagitis, and 12% had Barrett's esophagus. So, it is reassuring that more than 40% of patients were found to be normal; however, it is the other nearly 60% of patients who have a positive exam and may need further treatment.

The esophagus is a tubular structure that is about 20 to 25 centimeters (about 10 inches) long and is primarily made up of muscle. The inside of the tube is called the lumen, and it has a smooth lining called the mucosa, which is whitish in color. Below this is the junction between the esophagus and stomach where the mucosa changes in color and type. Stomach (gastric) mucosa is pink or salmon-colored and produces acid, among other things. At the bottom of the esophagus is the lower esophageal sphincter, or LES. The LES is a circular muscle located within the wall of the esophagus and closes to prevent reflux of material up from the stomach into the esophagus.

In an endoscopy, the scope travels down through the lumen of the esophagus to examine the mucosa. Irregularities easily can be seen and documented with photos or video and biopsies taken if needed. Esophagitis is inflammation of the esophageal mucosa caused by acid. Usually this occurs at the bottom near the stomach (gastric)–esophagus junction (called the GEJ). Esophagitis is graded on its severity and can range from mild, patchy redness of the mucosa to severe inflammation with loss of most of the esophageal mucosa with extensive ulceration.

*Chronic acid damage of the esophageal lining can result in recurrent inflammation with replacement of the normal mucosa with an acid-resistant abnormal mucosa called Barrett's esophagus.*

Chronic acid damage of the esophageal lining can result in recurrent inflammation with replacement of the normal mucosa with an acid-resistant abnormal mucosa called Barrett's esophagus. Endoscopically, this looks like tongues of salmon-colored mucosa extending from the gastroesophageal junction, **GEJ**, up into the esophagus. This area requires a biopsy to determine whether it has the microscopic features that confirm the diagnosis of Barrett's esophagus. Esophageal strictures or rings can be seen in patients with GERD, although generally these occur in patients with difficulty swallowing. Endoscopically, these range from a smooth, regular-appearing narrowing that easily allow passage of the scope, which is as wide as your pinkie, to a tight, ulcerated narrowing, which can be as small as a pinhole. These strictures can be biopsied, stretched, or dilated with or assisted by the endoscope. So, endoscopy is diagnostic and demonstrates whether a person has damage from chronic GERD, and it is therapeutic, allowing biopsy and treatment.

## 67. Who should have an endoscopy and why?

As mentioned, nearly 60% of people with chronic or frequent GERD have positive findings on endoscopy. Endoscopy is recommend for all patients with GERD symptoms longer than 6 months in duration and/or symptoms that occur 2 or more times per week.

Endoscopy serves as a baseline exam and enables your physician to determine whether there is active inflammation or damage and chronic changes that require treatment and further follow-up. Or you may be reassured that everything looks normal. Barrett's esophagus can be diagnosed and biopsied to ensure that there are no suspicious precancerous changes.

All patients who have difficulty swallowing should undergo endoscopy, which can provide clues to possible causes. It may be caused by a benign inflammatory stricture that can be dilated at the time of endoscopy or a malignant stricture that needs biopsy and further follow-up.

People at increased risk for esophageal or stomach cancer in addition to GERD should consider endoscopy. Those with a family history of esophageal or stomach cancer, smokers, and chronic alcohol users are at increased risk for cancer.

## 68. What is a manometry or motility study and why is it done?

Several different tests are available for evaluation of GERD and heartburn symptoms. Barium studies and endoscopy give your physician information about the structure of both a normal and abnormal esophagus and upper gastroesophageal tract. Sometimes if patients have atypical symptoms, do not respond appropriately to medications, or are under consideration for surgery, other tests may be in order.

During a normal swallow of food or liquid, muscles contract and relax in a very closely coordinated fashion. This contraction moves food or liquid from the

*During a normal swallow of food or liquid, muscles contract and relax in a very closely coordinated fashion.*

mouth down the esophagus to the stomach. This whole sequence allows you to swallow while you are upright or lying down and normally keeps material from refluxing from the stomach into the esophagus. On swallowing, material is pushed from the mouth into the upper esophagus and a valve, the **upper esophageal sphincter (UES),** opens. Then a contraction wave begins at the UES and pushes food down to the bottom of the esophagus and LES. When food reaches the LES, the LES relaxes, allowing food to enter the stomach. This is a very complicated process that remarkably takes only about 8 seconds.

A manometry or **motility study** is an exam that measures pressure in the stomach and esophagus. This permits an exam of the physiology of the esophagus and tells your physician whether the sphincters are relaxing and contracting at the appropriate times. It also gives information about whether the contraction wave is coordinated or in spasm and whether the waves are too weak or strong.

A **manometry study** is generally done at a center where endoscopy is performed, such as a hospital, ambulatory endoscopy center, or surgical center. It is generally performed without medication or sedation. A thin tube is passed into the nose or mouth, into the esophagus, and down to the stomach. The tube is about as thick as a piece of spaghetti. It is attached to several pressure sensors and it is very slowly pulled out while the patient is instructed to swallow either nothing or sips of water. The test allows many pressure readings in the stomach and throughout the esophagus. These data are then analyzed with a computer and a doctor goes over the results. This gives your physician an overall profile of the pressures within the esophagus and its response to swallowing. A motility study can help guide your doctor to more appropriate treatment, particularly for patients who do not respond to standard medication.

## 69. What is a pH study and why is it done?

The stomach makes acid that aids in digestion of food. GERD, or heartburn, is movement of the acid into the esophagus. Sometimes patients have vague, odd, or atypical symptoms instead of classic burning chest discomfort. A trial of antacid medication can help sort this out if your symptoms go away with treatment. But other things can cause chest pain like heart or lung problems and can be very difficult to differentiate from GERD. Additionally, patients with GERD symptoms may be on a maximum amount of medication and still experience GERD-type symptoms.

A pH study measures the amount of acid present in the esophagus and how long it stays there. This helps determine when a patient actually has pain or discomfort and the amount of acid in the esophagus to see if they correlate. When you experience heartburn and the pH test shows acid, then true GERD is present. But frequently people may have heartburn symptoms with no acid; this is not GERD, may need to be treated differently, and will not respond to antacid medication.

A pH study is usually done at an endoscopy center and occasionally may be performed at a doctor's office. It is generally done without sedation; a tiny probe is moved up the nose and down into the esophagus. The probe is connected to an **event recorder**, which looks like a pager. This recorder measures the amount of acid in

*When you experience heartburn and the pH test shows acid, then true GERD is present. But frequently people may have heart-burn symp-toms with no acid; this is not GERD, may need to be treated differ-ently, and will not respond to antacid med-ication.*

the esophagus and how long it stays there. You go home with this and return the next day. When you experience pain or heartburn, you push a button on the event recorder and the time is noted. The whole device (probe and monitor) is worn for about 24 hours. When you return to the doctor's office, the probe is easily removed and a computer analyzes the event recorder. This provides a lot of information such as how often in a 24-hour period your GERD occurs; how long it lasts when it does occur; and whether your subjective symptoms agree with the presence of acid reflux or not.

# PART EIGHT

# H. pylori, GERD, and Peptic Ulcer Disease

What is the relationship between ulcers and GERD?

Does gastroesophageal reflux disease cause ulcers?

Does *H. pylori* cause GERD?

*More...*

## 70. What is the relationship between ulcers and GERD?

An ulcer is a break in the lining of the gut generally defined as greater than 5 millimeters, which is about a quarter of an inch. Ulcers can occur anywhere in the gut from the mouth to the anus. The causes of ulcers vary depending on their location. Aspirin and nonsteroidal anti-inflammatory drugs (NSAIDs) such as ibuprofen and naproxen (Naprosyn) can cause ulcers anywhere in the gut. Classically, ulcers are located in the stomach and first part of the small intestine (called the duodenum). Aspirin, NSAIDs, infection of the stomach with the bacterium *H. pylori*, or the production of too much acid can cause these ulcers. Cigarette smoking can also play a role in ulcers and impair their healing.

Peptic ulcer disease (PUD) is the presence or history of ulcers of the stomach or duodenum. Some people with PUD have pain; typically this is a gnawing or burning discomfort in the middle of the upper abdomen that may improve with eating. There can be associated nausea, vomiting, poor appetite, and weight loss. Frequently, ulcers are silent and cause no pain or symptoms but may be discovered on an endoscopy.

*Typically, PUD is not associated with GERD.*

Typically, PUD is not associated with GERD. The confusion about this is because frequently patients with GERD can have the same or similar symptoms to that of someone with an ulcer. The treatment for PUD and GERD can be the same with H2 blockers or PPI medications. Additionally, when patients with GERD have endoscopy or barium studies, an ulcer in the esophagus is commonly found. This is not peptic ulcer disease. Esophageal ulcers are not caused by an *H. pylori* infection. Esophageal ulcers are caused by acid burning the area and or by certain medications. Examples of medications that cause esophageal ulcers are aspirin and NSAIDs, potassium pills, iron pills, medications for osteoporosis such as alendronate sodium, and certain antibiotics like tetracycline. This is a short list; there are many more, but these are the most common causes.

The only real relationship of PUD to GERD is acid. To get PUD the stomach needs to produce acid. Obviously, to have GERD you need acid refluxing up into the esophagus. This is the reason antacid medications are effective in treating both diseases.

## 71. Does gastroesophageal reflux disease cause ulcers?

As mentioned earlier, when people talk about ulcers, they usually are speaking of ulcers in the stomach or part of the small intestine, the duodenum. GERD does not cause this type of ulcer. Ulcers can occur in the esophagus, but through a different mechanism. Esophageal ulcers are generally caused by GERD when acid damages the lining of the esophagus. Esophageal ulcers can cause symptoms or can be silent and have no symptoms. The symptoms associated with an esophageal ulcer can be heartburn, difficulty swallowing with the feeling of food getting stuck, or pain on swallowing.

Richard's comment:

*I do not have ulcers or other stomach problems at this time. But by educating myself about a lot of the nasty issues that can arise in the digestive tract, I appreciate that some health problems are genetic whereas others are caused by our own actions. Although I cannot change my genetics, I sure can be smarter with how I live.*

## 72. *What is* H. pylori*?*

There really is no strong association between *H. pylori* infection and GERD. However, we discuss it here because invariably patients have questions about *H. pylori* infection and its association to disease, particularly to stomach problems. *H. pylori* is a bacterium or germ and is one of the most common infections in humans. It is present in about half of the world population. *H. pylori* is uncommon in children living in the developed world and is usually acquired as people age. In the United States, estimates suggest that approximately 40–50% of people have *H. pylori*. In underdeveloped countries with poor sanitation, lack of appropriate sewage systems, and inadequate water treatment facilities, *H. pylori* infection is common and occurs in childhood. In these countries, infection is present in greater than 75% of adults.

*In the United States, estimates suggest that approximately 40–50% of people have H. pylori.*

The spread or transmission of *H. pylori* has not been completely worked out. It is suggested that it is spread by the oral–oral or fecal–oral route. Oral-oral means from mouth to mouth, for example, sharing utensils or toothbrushes or drinking glasses. Fecal-oral means that somehow human waste gets into food or drink, for example, when human waste contaminates a water supply.

Most people with *H. pylori* infection have no symptoms, and not all people with *H. pylori* infections get ulcers or experience damage. *H. pylori* causes ulcers of the duodenum and stomach. It does not cause heartburn or GERD or ulcers of the esophagus. Sometimes *H. pylori* can cause stomach or duodenal irritation that can feel like a stomachache, gnawing discomfort, sour stomach, or nausea. More serious ulcer symptoms can be nausea, vomiting, weight loss, and even bleeding. Bleeding can be vomiting up blood or passing blood that looks black in the stool. This is a serious condition and requires an urgent visit to the nearest emergency room because it can be life-threatening.

The stomach produces acid that helps to digest food. Stomach acid is very strong and corrosive and can burn various tissues such as the esophagus. Special cells are in the stomach lining that make mucus protect the stomach from the acid that coats the stomach. *H. pylori* infects the stomach and duodenum, where it lives and grows in the protective mucus. *H. pylori* bacteria release toxins that kill or damage the mucus-producing cells. The loss of the mucous layer enables the acid to reach the stomach lining and cause damage that ultimately results in an ulcer. Further, this long-standing damage and repair of the stomach lining increases the risk of developing stomach cancer. There is a strong association between *H. pylori* and stomach cancer.

## 73. Does H. pylori *cause GERD?*

*H. pylori* does not really cause GERD. But some recent medical studies suggest that *H. pylori* infection can play a small role in heartburn. Because *H. pylori* damages the lining of the stomach, the stomach produces less acid. If acid production is decreased, in some people *H. pylori* infection may actually protect against GERD or at least decrease the amount of acid in the material that is refluxed from the stomach into the esophagus. So, if you have GERD and find out that you also have an *H. pylori* infection, getting the infection treated could make the GERD symptoms worse. However, given the risk of developing an ulcer or stomach cancer, the current recommendation is to treat the infection if it is diagnosed.

> H. pylori *does not really cause GERD.*

## 74. Do I need to be checked for H. pylori?

If you have GERD, the answer is no. If you have a history of stomach or duodenal ulcers even in the remote past, then yes, you should be checked. If you have a primary relative like a parent or brother or sister who has stomach cancer, then it is probably a good idea to be checked for *H. pylori* infection. Treating an *H. pylori* infection can decrease your chances of getting future ulcers and your risk for getting stomach cancer. In an endoscopy, if your physician finds any irritation of the stomach or duodenum or finds ulcers, then he or she should perform stomach biopsies to check for infection.

There is some debate, but it can be helpful to check for *H. pylori* in patients with dyspepsia. *Dyspepsia* is a nonspecific term for a sour stomach. Dyspepsia has many causes, and symptoms can be bloating, nausea, upper abdominal discomfort or pain, feeling filled up quickly while eating, vomiting, or indigestion. The diagnosis and treatment of *H. pylori* in people with these symptoms might be helpful. Often the treatment may not help with the dyspepsia symptoms. However, given the association of *H. pylori* to ulcers and cancer, it is not unreasonable to look for and treat infection with this bacteria in these patients.

## 75. What are the tests for H. pylori?

There are many ways to test for *H. pylori* infection, invasive tests and noninvasive tests. The most effective noninvasive test is called the urease breath test. Urea is a waste product humans make and excrete in the urine. Humans cannot digest or metabolize urea. *H. pylori* bacteria metabolize and use urea. Many of the tests for *H. pylori* are based on urea metabolism. In a **urease breath test**, you drink a small amount of very mildly radioactive urea, and then in a few minutes your breath is collected in a bag and analyzed. Normally, you breathe in oxygen and breathe out carbon dioxide. If radioactive carbon dioxide is present in the bag, then *H. pylori* is present and has digested the radioactive urea. This test is useful because it detects active infection.

There are also blood tests for *H. pylori*. Blood tests detect the presence of *H. pylori* antibodies in the blood. An antibody is a protein your body produces when you are exposed to a foreign substance, such as an infection. The problem with this test is when you've had a prior *H. pylori* infection that is gone, the test remains positive. Stool tests are also available to check for *H. pylori*.

Invasive tests are done at the time of an endoscopy. The stomach can be biopsied and checked for *H. pylori* infection. The tissue can be stained with special chemicals and examined under the microscope by a pathologist to look for the actual bacteria. Or a CLO test can be done, which is when a stomach biopsy is done and the tissue is placed in a tiny well containing a gel with urea in it. If *H. pylori* bacteria are present, they will metabolize the urea and the well will change color. These tests are very useful because they diagnose an active infection and not a previous one.

## 76. If I have *H. pylori*, should I be treated?

The general recommendation is yes. As mentioned, *H. pylori* causes peptic ulcer disease and is a risk factor for stomach cancer. Because of these risks treatment is recommended for patients with documented *H. pylori* infection. The treatment, however, is somewhat complicated. Usually, when a patient has an infection, such as a urinary tract infection, a course of a single antibiotic is given for a few days. But *H. pylori* is difficult to treat and requires multiple drugs in combination.

*Generally, the treatment for H. pylori involves an acid-controlling medication such as a PPI or H2 blocker in combination with two antibiotics and sometimes a bismuth-containing drug such as Pepto-Bismol.*

Generally, the treatment involves an acid-controlling medication such as a PPI or H2 blocker in combination with two antibiotics and sometimes a bismuth-containing drug such as Pepto-Bismol. These drugs are taken for 10 to 14 days. Sometimes these drugs are prescribed separately, or they can be given in a combination pack. For example, depending on drug allergies, Prevpac might be prescribed. This is a box of medication that contains lansoprazole (Prevacid), a proton pump inhibitor, amoxicillin, and clarithromycin, which are two antibiotics. Patients with an allergy to penicillin cannot take this because amoxicillin is a penicillin-like drug. Another combination drug regimen for *H. pylori* is bismuth with two antibiotics, metronidazole and tetracycline (Helidac). This is prescribed with an antiacid medication such as ranitidine. These combination therapies cost $200 to $300 and are covered by most drug prescription insurance plans.

There are risks to treatment because all medications have side effects. Most antibiotics can causecan develop to any of the combined medications stomach upset or diarrhea. Also, an allergy to any of the combined medications can develop.

# PART NINE

# Medications for Gastroesophageal Reflux Disease

What are antacids and how and when should they be used?

What are the differences between H2 blockers and proton pump inhibitors?

What should I do if the medication is not working?

*More...*

## 77. What are antacids, and how and when should they be used?

Antacids are compounds that can be used to neutralize acid on the spot, thus providing immediate relief of heartburn symptoms. Antacids are available at any drugstore, convenience store, and supermarket. All antacid products are over the counter and do not require a prescription. They are available for the general consumer to use at his or her own discretion. As mentioned, more than 7 million people suffer from regular GERD, and even more people suffer from occasional or infrequent heartburn symptoms. For this reason, people can choose from the hundreds of available options for antacids. They are available in many different forms: tablets, chewable pills, liquids, elixirs, or even powders that can be dissolved in water and ingested. Antacid products are available for adults and child use. The main purpose of all of these medications is to provide a substance that can block the damaging effects of acid that causes reflux symptoms.

To understand how antacids work, a short chemistry lesson is in order. There are acids (such as stomach acid, the acid in car batteries, or even foods like vinegar), and the opposite of these compounds are called bases (such as baking soda or strong bases such as Drano, which is used to clean pipes). Depending on the environment, which can be either acidic or basic. However, if you mix an acid and base in equal proportions, you can create a neutral environment. Thus, the antacid, a basic compound, works by neutralizing acid in the esophagus and stomach, making the refluxed fluid bland and no longer damaging. A classic example (and one you can try easily) is to take vinegar, an acid, and mix it with baking soda, a base. The result is a

*Antacids are compounds that can be used to neutralize acid on the spot, thus providing immediate relief of heartburn symptoms.*

chemical reaction that produces bubbling and gas. This is sort of what happens in your stomach when you take an antacid. Some antacid preparations put on this "show" before you even take them, for example, when you place an **Alka Seltzer** tablet in a glass of water.

Antacids are generally used as first-line therapy for mild heartburn symptoms that occur occasionally. However, many people use antacids inappropriately, for example, the frequent heartburn sufferer who has symptoms many times a day and walks around eating an entire roll of calcium carbonate (Tums) or calcium carbonate and magnesium hydroxide (Rolaids) each day. Antacids are more effective and beneficial for those who experience reflux sporadically or less than once a week. H2 blockers and proton pump inhibitors are much more effective if you have regular symptoms several times a week or daily because these drugs prevent acid production. Generally speaking, antacids do not prevent reflux symptoms from occurring, rather they treat symptoms after they have occurred.

*Generally speaking, antacids do not prevent reflux symptoms from occurring, rather they treat symptoms after they have occurred.*

As discussed, antacids come in many formulations, meaning they contain many different active ingredients to neutralize acid. Some are more effective than others and also may have other added health benefits or side effects. A favorite antacid that I use regularly (DLB) is calcium carbonate. Calcium carbonate comes in many flavors, is chewable, and is effective for GERD. But an added benefit of calcium carbonate is that it contains calcium. Adults require 1200 to 1600 milligrams of calcium per day to maintain bone health, and this can be easily achieved by taking a few calcium carbonate tablets each day. In fact, I frequently recommend that my patients take calcium carbonate as a calcium supplement even if they do not have GERD.

In summary, antacids do not decrease production of stomach acid but rather neutralize acid and decrease symptoms of reflux. Antacids are most effective for those with infrequent reflux to treat symptoms as they occur, not to prevent them.

## 78. Antacids seem benign. Do they have side effects?

Antacids are medications, and even though they are available without a prescription, you should be advised that they too can cause side effects and have adverse effects. Antacids are drugs that contain multiple ingredients in addition to the active agent that neutralizes acid. There are dyes for coloring, flavors, fillers to form the actual tablet or pill, and other additives. Any one of these can cause problems in certain people.

*Antacids are medications, and even though they are available without a prescription, you should be advised that they too could cause side effects and have adverse effects.*

Some antacids are mixed with aspirin to act as a pain reliever, for example, Alka Seltzer. As noted previously, aspirin can also cause stomach irritation and generally should be avoided in those with bad reflux disease. Aspirin can increase risks of ulcers or bleeding and should not be mixed with certain medications such as warfarin.

Other antacids are composed with sodium, a salt that is bound to the base used to neutralize the acid. The inadvertent ingestion of extra sodium can cause fluid retention. Many people with high blood pressure and/or a heart condition called congestive heart failure are on low-sodium diets. Consumption of sodium-containing antacids can increase blood pressure or aggravate heart failure in predisposed individuals.

Some antacids are mixed with calcium or magnesium as a binding agent for the base that is used to neutralize acid. These two elements can cause different side effects with respect to the bowels. The easily absorbed calcium can cause constipation. On the other hand, the magnesium is poorly absorbed and can cause diarrhea. A hint you can use to distinguish whether the antacid contains magnesium is that most magnesium-containing antacids begin with the letter *M* such as Maalox (aluminum) or Mylanta (magnesium/simethicone). Milk of magnesia and magnesium citrate, two potent laxatives used to help alleviate constipation, contain magnesium because magnesium is a great laxative.

Antacids can interact with other medications, and it is important to read the label of any medications you are taking to see if antacids should be avoided. To work, some medications require acid and taking an antacid may reduce their activity or effects. Others interact directly with agents in the antacids. Again, examples are the calcium-containing antacids. Some antibiotics used to treat infection interact with calcium and should not be taken at the same time as antacids. Commonly used medication for high blood pressure called calcium channel blockers also interact with calcium-containing antacids and should be avoided.

Fillers or binders are compounds added to medications so that they can be pressed into a tablet or can dissolve appropriately. Sugars commonly added to drugs can be a source of added calories if taken in large quantities. **Sorbitol** is a sugar that adds sweetness without calories that is occasionally added to pills, but it can also be a laxative and cause diarrhea. Lactose is another sugar binder that can cause gas, bloating, and diarrhea in those with lactose intolerance.

The preceding are only a few examples of side effects and drug–drug interactions. It is very important to read labels on both your medications and antacids. If you are not sure, your pharmacist will know or can look up the drug interactions or adverse effects.

## 79. If antacids do not work or are not appropriate for my GERD, what is the next step or tier of medications to try?

Antacids are first-line therapy for mild or infrequent heartburn; however, sometimes these medications will not work or are simply not appropriate. To properly understand the other options available for anti-reflux therapy, it is important to know the biology of the stomach and how it produces acid for digestion.

*Multiple factors can stimulate production of stomach acid.*

The stomach has multiple actions that aid in digestion of food. The stomach stores food and, with strong muscles, grinds food material into pieces less than a half inch in size. Simultaneously, fluid, acid, and digestive enzymes are secreted by the stomach lining into the mix, which starts the process of digestion. Multiple factors can stimulate production of stomach acid. The sight, smell, or taste of food will "get the juices flowing," as will the presence of food within the stomach, which distends it. These events stimulate the brain to release different substances such as hormones that target stomach lining cells (**parietal cells**) to make acid. One substance made by nerves controlling acid production is called **histamine**.

You may commonly use an antihistamine; these medications are for allergies and sometimes colds. Allergic reactions such as hay fever with a stuffy nose, watery or itchy eyes, itchy skin, rash, and coughing are caused by extra histamine production. So, by blocking the action of histamine with an antihistamine, you block its action.

Stomach acid cells are sensitive to histamine and when exposed to histamine are stimulated to produce acid. Regular antihistamines such as those for allergies do not work on the stomach. However, a different kind of histamine blocker called a histamine-2 blocker (H2 blocker) is effective at decreasing stomach acid production.

When the stomach acid cells are stimulated by histamine, they turn on special microscopic pumps within the cell called proton pumps. These proton pumps secrete acid into the stomach. Another class of drugs available to block acid production is called proton pump inhibitors (PPIs).

*H2 blockers and PPIs reduce/eliminate stomach acid... These medications treat GERD before it happens and prevent it.*

To recap, there are several ways to stimulate stomach acid production and two effective classes of medications, called H2 blockers and proton pump inhibitors, or PPIs. The benefit of these drugs is they reduce or eliminate stomach acid and are very effective for the treatment of GERD or peptic ulcer disease (stomach or duodenal ulcers). Thus, these medications treat GERD before it happens and prevent it.

There are many differences between H2 blockers and PPIs, including effectiveness, cost, side effects, and dosing. Because of these issues, H2 blockers are considered second-tier drugs after antacids. If H2 blockers fail, third-tier medications are PPIs.

## 80. What are the differences between H2 blockers and proton pump inhibitors? What are the H2 blockers? How are they dosed and taken, and are they expensive?

H2 blockers reduce acid production, whereas PPIs block acid production altogether. So, PPIs are considered much stronger. Many H2 blockers are available, and most are over the counter (OTC) and do not require a doctor's prescription. They come in generic or plain forms that are cheaper than the proprietary or marketed forms of the same drug. For the most part, both forms of the drugs work about the same, and for mild to moderate GERD the generics are a cost savings and work fine. There are four H2 blockers available in the United States and are sold under several names. Table 4 lists the available medications in alphabetical order.

*H2 blockers reduce acid production, whereas PPIs block acid production altogether.*

Some OTC H2 blockers are marketed at half of the usual prescription strength; it is important to read the

**Table 4    H2 Blocker Medications**

| Medication (generic) | Medication (trade) | Doses | Approx. prices (Drugstore.com) |
|---|---|---|---|
| Cimetidine | Tagamet | 300 mg. twice a day | $16 to $70 for 60 pills |
| Famotidine | Pepcid, Fluxid | 20 to 40 mg twice a day | $19 to $100 for 30 pills |
| Nizatidine | Axid | 75 to 150 mg twice a day | $10 to $160 for 30 pills |
| Ranitidine | Zantac | 75 to 150 mg twice a day | $8 to $140 for 60 pills |

label to see the strength and dose. The prices in the table are approximate and are included only to show you that the generics are dramatically cheaper than the proprietary drugs. The dosing given is average or usual dosing; the actual dosing for GERD could be less or more depending on the severity of your GERD, so read the dosing recommendations on the package label. As mentioned, these are all available without a prescription, but many nonprescription drugs are not covered under most prescription drug insurance plans. Higher dosing may be available with a doctor's prescription and could be medications covered by insurance. In most states, there is usually a mandatory substitution to a generic drug if you use a doctor's prescription.

H2 blockers are effective for mild to moderate GERD symptoms. These drugs have been shown in medical studies to be effective in healing esophagitis (inflammation of the lining of the esophagus). And once healed, H2 blockers are effective in maintaining healing of esophagitis when used long-term.

H2 blockers come as pills and a few as elixirs or liquids. After you take the pills, an H2 blocker takes about an hour to start working. So, an antacid might be a better choice if your reflux has already started. Some OTC H2 blockers such as famotidine/calcium carbonate/magnesium hydroxide (Pepcid Complete) come with an antacid included, are effective immediately, and can last up to 12 hours.

For those with predictable, occasional GERD, the medication should be taken before symptoms occur. For example, if you are going out for spicy food and are going to have a few alcoholic drinks, take an H2 blocker prior to the meal. If you only have nighttime GERD, then take medication before bed. If you have GERD daily and several times a day, then take a full dose daily to be more effective. Most H2 blockers reduce acid production for 6 to 12 hours and, accordingly, depending on the particular drug, you can take them anywhere from two to four times a day.

H2 blockers have been on the market for more than 25 years and before PPIs were developed were the number one prescribed drug in the United States. Millions of people have safely used these medications for years, and they are very safe for long-term use. But H2 blockers may not offer enough acid suppression for everyone. Those with severe GERD, asthma, aspiration, esophageal strictures, or Barrett's esophagus may need complete elimination of stomach acid. Proton pump inhibitors are more effective for severe GERD and its complications.

## 81. What are the different proton pump inhibitors? How should they be taken?

*Proton pump inhibitors completely shut down stomach cells that produce acid because they work directly on the site of acid production.*

Proton pump inhibitors completely shut down stomach cells that produce acid because they work directly on the site of acid production. Because they are the strongest acid-blocking medication, they are considered third-tier treatment for GERD. The tiers represent the step-wise management of GERD symptoms, starting with the cheapest and safest medication as first tier and ending with PPIs as third tier. PPIs are the most expensive medications for GERD and have, generally speaking, more side effects.

**Table 5   PPI Medications**

| Generic Name | Proprietary Name | Usual Dose | Cost (drugstore.com) |
|---|---|---|---|
| Esomeprazole | Nexium | 40 mg once or twice a day | 40 mg 30 pills $124 |
| Lansoprazole | Prevacid | 30 mg once or twice a day | 30 mg 30 pills $124 |
| Omeprazole | Prilosec, Prilosec OTC, Zegerid | 20 to 40 mg once or twice a day | 20 mg pack $132** |
| Pantoprazole | Protonix | 40 mg once or twice a day | 40 mg 30 pills $111 |
| Rabeprazole | Aciphex | 20 mg once or twice a day | 20mg 30 pills $122 |

**please a see above for comment on generic prices

Currently, only one over-the-counter PPI, Prilosec OTC, is available; all others require a prescription. (see Table 5). Omeprazole is available only by prescription. A lot of this is marketing by the drug companies because Prilosec OTC (20-mg pills) costs about $13 for 14 pills and generic prescription omeprazole (20-mg pills) costs about $42 for 14 pills. Despite the previous comment that proprietary and generic drugs are about the same, in my experience (DLB), Prilosec OTC is a much more effective drug and costs a quarter as much as the generic.

*Prilosec OTC is a much more effective drug and costs a quarter as much as the generic.*

Proton pump inhibitors as a group are overall much more effective for controlling stomach acid production than H2 blockers are. Proton pump inhibitors are the drug of choice for severe GERD symptoms, esophagitis, strictures, and Barrett's esophagus. Sometimes PPIs are used to heal esophageal damage, and then patients are switched to an H2 blocker for long-term maintenance. In many studies, proton pump inhibitors have been shown to be more effective than H2 blockers are in healing esophagitis and maintaining healing. And if symptoms cannot be controlled with an H2 blocker, then long-term PPIs are continued.

Despite the fact that PPIs are strong, they are virtually useless if heartburn is already present because PPIs can take hours to a day to start working. These drugs are most effectively used to prevent GERD from occurring. So, PPIs should be taken regularly once or twice a day, not just on the spot when heartburn occurs. A common misconception among patients who take PPIs is that they feel the drug does not work, when really they are taking it incorrectly. Further, PPIs are very sensitive and do not work effectively if you do not take them at the appropriate time. *All PPIs must be taken 30 to 45 minutes before eating food.* This recommendation cannot be stressed enough. Many patients take PPIs when they get up in the morning, and then they do not eat breakfast, or they take the medication at bedtime for nighttime GERD—this is incorrect. If the drug is taken once a day, it should be a half hour before breakfast. If a PPI is taken twice a day, the additional dose is taken half an hour before dinner. Taking a PPI appropriately will ensure you get the maximum benefit from the medication.

*PPIs are very sensitive and do not work effectively if you do not take them at the appropriate time. All PPIs must be taken 30 to 45 minutes before eating food.*

Proton pump inhibitors have been on the market in the United States for more than 15 years and have been used by millions of patients. The original drug omeprazole was the number one prescribed drug in the United States for years. Omeprazole and other PPIs are safe and effective for long-term use.

Richard's comment:

*Currently, I am taking a PPI called pantoprazole, (Protonix) 40 mg. It has worked well for me, but I recently realized it should be taken 30 to 45 minutes before my evening meal. Up until then, I was taking it in the morning. I do not eat breakfast, so this was a mistake. Pantoprazole should work even better now that I am taking it at the correct time of day.*

## 82. What are the major side effects associated with H2 blockers and PPIs?

All medications have benefits and risks. Unfortunately, the side effects of a prescription or OTC drug cannot always be predicted or prevented. In certain people, however rare, these medications can cause side effects. The side effects are very similar between the two classes of medications discussed here, and the effects seem to be dose dependent: with higher doses comes an increased risk of potential side effects.

H2 blockers and proton pump inhibitors (PPIs) act primarily on the digestive system, and for this reason, the majority of the potential side effects tend to involve the stomach and digestion. In approximately 5% of patients, both classes of medications can cause nausea, abdominal pain, diarrhea, and even constipation. Diarrhea is most closely associated with PPI use and occurs in about 5–10% of people. Periodically, patients have had to discontinue their PPI use because of diarrhea.

The drugs are absorbed into your bloodstream and circulate throughout the body, so the effects are not limited to the stomach and esophagus. These effects are usually mild and tend to resolve with time. In other cases, the side effects can be severe enough to warrant stopping the medication. These medications have also been reported to cause headaches. Particularly, those who have frequent migraines may have increased headache symptoms.

There is some variability in the side effects and potency of different PPIs. If a mild but problematic side effect occurs, try another PPI. However, rare and serious reactions have occurred, including life-threatening allergic reactions. Allergic reactions to H2 blockers and PPIs are very rare and include rashes, itching, wheezing, swelling, or difficulty breathing. If you have any question about an allergic reaction, immediately discontinue the medication and avoid the entire class of medication in the future. The drugs within a class, either PPIs or H2 blockers, are similar and an allergic reaction to one specific drug can be a sign of allergy to the entire class of drugs.

Dangerous side effects include decreasing blood counts, decreasing platelet counts, confusion, and liver damage (see Table 6). These effects can happen at any time in the course of taking an H2 blocker or PPI. In these cases, immediately stop taking the medication and discuss the side effects with your doctor.

Richard's comment:

*I have been on pantoprazole, (Protonix) 40 mg for about 6 months. I haven't experienced any major or serious side effects from the medication thus far.*

**Table 6  Side Effects of H2 Blockers and Proton Pump Inhibitors**

| H2 blockers | Proton Pump Inhibitors |
|---|---|
| Constipation | Headache |
| Diarrhea | Diarrhea |
| Headache | Constipation |
| Nausea | Abdominal pain |
| Vomiting | |
| Confusion | |
| Dizziness | |
| Drop in blood counts | |
| Drop in platelet counts | |
| Dry mouth or skin | |
| Hair loss | |
| Decrease in libido | |
| Breast or chest soreness | |
| Rash | |

## 83. How should I take the medications, and when will they work?

As discussed earlier, different medications have different mechanisms of action to treat reflux. Antacids are most effective during a bout of reflux because they directly neutralize the acid. But they do not prevent reflux and only last for brief periods of time.

Second-tier therapies, H2 blockers, are safe and are best taken before reflux occurs. For example, a person with nighttime GERD might take a bedtime dose of an H2 blocker. If you have occasional GERD and plan to have a spicy meal, then taking a dose prior to the meal (as needed) may be better. Those with more frequent or severe symptoms can take a full dose of medication daily. Most H2 blockers are taken two, three, or rarely, four times a day.

*Proton pump inhibitors work by a different mechanism and are very ineffective for treating GERD that is already occurring. These medications take 24 to 48 hours to start working. PPIs need to be taken at the appropriate time for maximum effect.*

Proton pump inhibitors work by a different mechanism and are very ineffective for treating GERD that is already occurring. These medications take 24 to 48 hours to start working. PPIs need to be taken at the appropriate time for maximum effect.

Proton pump inhibitors are most effective before a meal. The pill is taken and absorbed into the bloodstream, and then travels back to act on the acid-producing cells of the stomach. The drug can then block the pump that is primed and ready to release acid as soon as it is stimulated by any food that enters the mouth or stomach. *Proton pump inhibitors have maximum strength if taken 30 minutes before food.* Most PPIs last for 10 to 18 hours and are taken once or twice a day.

## 84. Do I need to take the medication every day or just when I have reflux?

The answer to this question depends on which medication you are taking. Antacids are used for temporary relief and have short-lived effects. Antacids are not generally taken every day but on an as-needed basis.

H2 blockers can be taken daily or before reflux occurs and usually take about an hour to start working. famotidine/calcium carbonate/magnesium hydroxide (Pepcid Complete) is a combination antacid and H2 blocker that offers immediate relief of reflux and up to 12 hours of acid suppression.

H2 blockers and PPIs are recommended for frequent symptoms that may be long-standing. This prolonged acid contact time can lead to complications such as strictures or Barrett's esophagus. Improvement of symptomatic esophagitis requires a two-phased approach. Initially, you must heal the acid-induced injury. Then once healed, you enter a maintenance phase to prevent recurrent damage. Most people who start regular use of an acid-suppressing medication stay on it for years, possibly for life.

Given the chronic nature of GERD, these drugs are taken at least daily and not sporadically. The only way to change this is by modifying your lifestyle or, if symptoms are debilitating, having anti-reflux surgery. These issues should be discussed with your doctor.

## 85. What should I do if the medication is not working?

You may not find over-the-counter H2 blockers effective for moderate to severe heartburn. If the reflux disease is severe enough, it may require increased medication dosing or a prescription-strength H2 blocker. If H2 blockers are not effective enough in controlling symptoms, then movement to the next tier of GERD therapy is warranted. PPIs are the most potent of the

*If the reflux disease is severe enough, it may require increased medication dosing or a prescription-strength H2 blocker.*

medications used to treat acid reflux because they block stomach acid production completely.

Remember, both H2 blockers and PPIs are very effective in preventing heartburn. They do not work well once symptoms have occurred—antacids are more effective when symptoms are present. If symptoms occur while you are taking an H2 blocker, read the label on the H2 blocker because not all drugs are sold at the same dose. Ranitidine HCL, for example, is sold over the counter and comes in a 75-mg and 150-mg pill. The packaging on both is nearly identical, and failure of the smaller dose may be remedied by taking the larger dose. Further, ranitidine HCL works for about 12 hours, if you have nighttime symptoms and are taking a dose at breakfast time, it will be ineffective because the medication ideally should be taken about an hour before anticipated symptoms. So, the strength of a medication and when it is taken account for most treatment failures. If these changes do not control symptoms, then a stronger medication may be in order.

The most common reason PPIs fail to work effectively is because they are taken incorrectly. As previously discussed, PPIs need to be in the bloodstream and available to cells that produce acid when the cells are ready to make acid. *PPIs do not work unless this is the case, and so must be taken 30 minutes prior to eating food.* Food stimulates the tiny pumps in stomach acid cells to make the actual acid. PPIs block this acid production by blocking the functioning of the proton pumps in the acid-producing cells. Pumps are only activated when acid production is stimulated and are inactive during periods when food is not available. So, the timing of taking PPIs must be closely coordinated with eating.

Most PPIs take 24 to 48 hours to work and may not work the first day you use them. Generally, PPIs work for 10 to 16 hours, so again, a pill taken before breakfast may not be effective for nighttime symptoms. Thus, if you have only nighttime GERD, a dose of PPI before dinner is more effective. Alternatively, if you have day and night symptoms, taking the medication twice a day, once before breakfast and once before dinner, may be more effective.

If the symptoms still do not resolve with twice-a-day dosing of the PPI, it may be time to discuss with your doctor the possibility of changing medications. Some PPIs are stronger than others, and trials of different drugs may help you find the most effective one. Finally, if all else fails, then more testing could be in order to confirm that your symptoms really are GERD and not something else such as a heart problem. On rare occasions, PPIs can fail to control GERD and a surgical anti-reflux procedure should be considered.

## 86. If my symptoms get better, can I stop taking medication?

It is reassuring to know that symptoms can respond to medication therapy. However, if your symptoms get dramatically better on prescription medication, it is important you continue this medication for a course of time, or at least until your doctor evaluates you again.

As previously discussed, medications work in two ways: they heal acid damage and they maintain healing. Generally speaking, it takes about 8 weeks to heal esophagitis, and the maintenance phase can last from months to years. Once you stop taking the medication, the whole process of damaging the esophagus by acid can reoccur. Because of this fact, many patients cannot stop their medications because reflux symptoms will return. Frequently, H2 blockers or PPIs need to be taken for life. The only way to change this is to modify your lifestyle. For example, overweight patients with GERD frequently experience improvement of symptoms and can decrease or stop medications when they lose weight. Cutting down or eliminating alcohol use and not eating for at least 2 hours prior to sleep can also help reduce medication requirements.

# PART TEN

# Endoscopic and Surgical Options for GERD

If my GERD is chronic and possibly lifelong, do I need to take medications for life or are there any other options?

What are the surgeries for GERD?

What are the long-term risks/benefits of endoscopic anti-reflux procedures?

*More...*

## 87. If my GERD is chronic and possibly lifelong, do I need to take medications for life or are there any other options?

If you have long-standing frequent GERD and lifestyle modifications such as weight loss do not improve your symptoms, then you may need to take medications for life. The good news is that H2 blockers are safe for long-term use and have been on the market for more than 25 years demonstrating their safety. Proton pump inhibitors are felt to be safe for long-term use as well, and these have been on the market for more than 15 years. There were early concerns with long-term PPI use because initial studies showed increased risk of a rare cancer in rats on omeprazole. However, these cancers never developed in humans taking long-term PPIs. Long-standing use of PPIs has sometimes been associated with development of a vitamin $B_{12}$ deficiency. A simple blood test by your doctor can check whether you have a $B_{12}$ deficiency. Also, people who take long-term PPIs have an increased risk of stomach polyps. Stomach polyps are benign polyps that do not turn into cancer; they are different from colon polyps, which do have cancerous potential.

*If you have long-standing frequent GERD and lifestyle modifications such as weight loss do not improve your symptoms, then you may need to take medications for life.*

You have other options to taking medications for life. Operations or procedures can be done endoscopically to tighten or strengthen your lower esophageal sphincter and improve reflux. These procedures can control reflux of acidic material and improve regurgitation. After these procedures you might be able to stop or reduce your GERD medication.

## 88. Should I have surgery for my GERD?

This is a difficult question to answer, and the decision really is yours. The real issue is how bad your GERD and/or regurgitation is. Does medication control your symptoms adequately? How difficult or costly is it to take a medication once or twice a day? Is your GERD making your life difficult or miserable? If the answer to these questions is yes, then surgery may be an option.

The goal of anti-reflux surgery is to strengthen the lower esophageal sphincter, which is the barrier to reflux of material from the stomach into the esophagus. First, there are risks to surgery and anesthesia— are you a surgical candidate? Because GERD can be treated with medication, this is elective surgery, meaning that the surgery is being done to improve your lifestyle, not for a life-and-death condition. Patients with heart disease such as angina, recent heart attacks, and congestive heart failure are at increased risk in surgery and under anesthesia. Those with severe lung disease such as asthma, chronic obstructive pulmonary disease (COPD), emphysema, or those on home oxygen are also at great risk. Obesity additionally increases the risks and makes wound healing and postoperative infections more likely. So, if you have any of the preceding conditions, surgery may not be right for you.

Prior to surgery an evaluation of the esophagus needs to be done. Before you are referred to a surgeon, have an endoscopy done to see if you have Barrett's esophagus or esophagitis. All patients are trialed on a proton pump inhibitor to see if preventing acid entering the esophagus makes their GERD symptoms better. Because not all burning chest discomfort is heartburn and because it is important to make sure the symptoms you are experiencing are truly GERD, you'll need a pH study to determine whether the pain or discomfort you have correlates to the presence of acid in your esophagus. You should also have a motility study to see whether your lower esophageal sphincter is weak or relaxes inappropriately and whether the rest of the esophagus pumps normally. Some diseases weaken both the LES and the muscles in the body of the esophagus that push food down to the stomach when you swallow. These are diagnosed with a motility study. If weakened LES and esophageal muscles are present and not found prior to surgery, you might not be able to swallow after surgery.

Any surgery carries risks. Patients can experience heart or lung problems from the stress of the operation or anesthesia. Bleeding or infections can complicate or prolong hospital stays. Patients can develop blood clots from the operation or from bed rest, and the clots can be life-threatening. Damage can be done to the stomach or esophagus during surgery. Not too uncommonly, surgery might make the lower esophageal sphincter too tight, and then patients have difficulty swallowing and need endoscopy and dilation. Some patients may require antacid medication again after surgery.

*Because of all of these issues and risks of surgery, we do not recommend anti-reflux surgery to many patients.*

Because of all of these issues and risks of surgery, we do not recommend anti-reflux surgery to many patients. It is usually reserved for young, healthy people that do not want to take lifelong medications or have severe, poorly controlled GERD symptoms on medications.

## 89. What are the surgeries for GERD?

There are two major ways to gain access to the abdomen: open operations and laparoscopic operations. In a classic operation, the surgeon uses a knife (scalpel) to make an incision and open the abdomen. Today, more surgeons are trained in laparoscopic surgery, which is a different technique that enables a surgeon to use a scope or camera to perform the surgery. This is different than an endoscope or endoscopy. For both open and laparoscopic surgery, the patient is brought to the operating room and put to sleep by the anesthesiologist. Laparoscopic surgery is done by making three to five small incisions (less that an inch long) around the abdomen and belly button. A wand-like camera is inserted through one of the incisions, and then the abdomen is inflated with gas so that the surgeon can have a view of all the organs on a television screen. The surgeon can then insert different long, thin tools through each of the other incisions to perform the operation.

Laparoscopic surgery is common today and is regularly used to remove gallbladders and do gastric bypass surgery for obesity and anti-reflux surgery. The benefits of doing laparoscopic versus open surgery are hospital stays are shorter, the surgical wounds are smaller, recovery is much quicker, and the risk of developing a hernia at the surgical site is lower.

Once inside the abdomen, anti-reflux surgery is roughly the same for both techniques. The most commonly performed anti-reflux procedure is called a

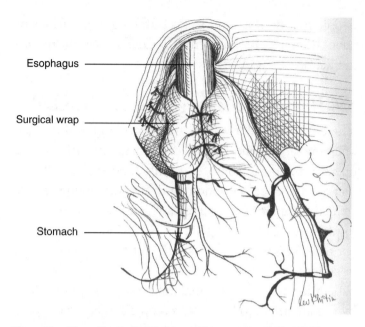

Esophagus

Surgical wrap

Stomach

**Figure 14    Nissen Fundoplication.** Source: Courtesy of Lev M. Khitin, MD.

**Nissen fundoplication** (see Figure 14). A Nissen procedure again can be done openly or laparoscopically and basically involves wrapping the top of the stomach all the way around the bottom of the esophagus to tighten the LES. There are several variations of this procedure; in one, the stomach is only partially wrapped around the bottom of the esophagus, and this is called a Toupet procedure. A Belsey Mark IV procedure is a partial wrap, but instead of going in through the abdomen, the surgeon goes in through the chest to get to the bottom of the esophagus. The end result of all of these procedures is to reinforce the lower esophageal sphincter, the barrier to reflux.

## 90. What are the long-term benefits and risks of surgery?

The benefits are control or elimination of GERD, regurgitation, and aspiration. Another benefit is the ability to stop taking or to reduce GERD medications possibly for life. Finally, surgery can lead to improvement in asthma or extraesophageal GERD symptoms.

Any operation and anesthesia is risky. A specific risk associated with anti-reflux surgery is resulting difficulty swallowing with food getting stuck. This can require endoscopy and dilation for treatment. Normally, you can belch and relieve excess gas; but patients who have had anti-reflux surgery can have abdominal bloating because they cannot belch. Diarrhea is not uncommon because the surgery may speed up stomach emptying. The ability to vomit can be impaired or it can become impossible in patients who have had an anti-reflux procedure. Hernias can develop within the abdomen or at the surgical wound site that can require repeat operation. Studies have demonstrated that more than 50% of patients who have had a Nissen procedure develop new and different symptoms postoperatively.

Historically, open Nissen fundoplications had a fixed lifespan, and after about 7 years the stitches holding the stomach together around the esophagus fell apart, requiring repeat operation. On rare occasions, the whole wrap, which should be in the abdomen, can herniate (move) into the chest and require another operation.

A French study by Pessaux and colleagues, published in 2005 in the *Archives of Surgery*, followed for 5 or more years 1340 patients who had anti-reflux surgery. The study found that about 5% of patients had severe difficulty with swallowing, more than 7% had gas and bloating, more than 5% of patients required another operation, and 10% of patients required a proton pump inhibitor to control GERD symptoms. Interestingly, in this study nearly 2700 patients had surgery, but less than half were available for study. This suggests that the patients who were happy with their surgery outcomes participated in the study, which skews the results to look better than they actually are. Also, the authors of the study were the surgeons who did the surgery.

This points out the problem of looking at the anti-reflux surgery literature: most of it is written by surgeons who perform the operation, and it may be biased.

## 91. Will I be able to stay off GERD medications if I have surgery?

Few studies have addressed this question. Short-term studies (2 years after surgery) show that surgery decreases the risk of esophagitis on endoscopy and improves GERD symptoms when compared to those patients who only take medications. However, medications are effective for alleviating both symptoms and esophagitis. A long-term study by Spechler and associates that was published in 1992 in the *New England Journal of Medicine* looked at patients 9 to 10 years after anti-reflux surgery and compared them to patients treated only with medication. The authors found that more than 60% of those who had the operation required medication for GERD in the long term. This study was done by gastroenterologists who treat GERD and may be more objective about surgical results than surgeons can be.

The previously mentioned French study showed that at 5 years after surgery, nearly 10% of patients required

*Short-term studies (2 years after surgery) show that surgery decreases the risk of esophagitis on endoscopy and improves GERD symptoms when compared to those patients who only take medications.*

a proton pump inhibitor. The authors did not comment on the need for other anti-acid medications such as H2 blockers.

So, the data suggest that surgery is effective in the short term, for a couple years, and helps improve GERD symptoms and esophagitis and decreases the need for medication. But in the long term, some patients will require medication for GERD.

## 92. Will surgery make my Barrett's esophagus improve or go away?

Again, not many studies address this question. Historically, in the medical literature, it was felt that surgery did not improve Barrett's esophagus. However, some recent small studies suggest that a slight improvement in Barrett's esophagus may occur after anti-reflux surgery. Overall, the current recommendation is that anti-reflux surgery is not effective treatment for Barrett's esophagus.

## 93. Will surgery decrease my risk of getting Barrett's-associated esophageal cancer?

There really is no data in the medical literature to answer this question. Of all patients with chronic GERD, 10% have Barrett's esophagus, and the risk of getting esophageal cancer with Barrett's is 0.5% per year (in other words, if 2000 people have GERD, 1 person per year will get esophageal cancer). Really, the risk of getting cancer with chronic GERD is low but is increased compared to those without GERD. For example, of those 2000 people previously mentioned,

80 will get colorectal cancer and 100 women will get breast cancer. Cancer risks need to be kept in perspective. So, the short answer is anti-reflux surgery will not decrease your risk of getting cancer associated with GERD and Barrett's esophagus.

## 94. How do I find a surgeon?

The most important issue in finding a surgeon for anti-reflux surgery is evaluating the surgeon's experience. (This really applies to any surgery.) Many studies have shown that more surgeon experience is associated with better results in surgery. You would not have heart bypass surgery performed by a surgeon who does one bypass a year—you want a heart surgeon who performs the operation every day or at least a couple times per week. This applies to reflux, too; the more anti-reflux operations a surgeon does in a year, the better. Because of this fact, you may benefit more by seeing a surgeon at a larger medical center or teaching hospital than by seeing one at a community hospital. Teaching hospitals are bigger, accept more difficult cases, and perform larger volumes of surgery. Community hospitals tend to have general surgeons who operate on many conditions—they remove gallbladders, remove colon cancers, remove breast cancers, and may do anti-reflux surgery once or twice a year. Because teaching hospitals are larger, surgeons can specialize in particular areas such as stomach surgery.

Younger surgeons have been trained in laparoscopic techniques; this is a relatively new technology. For example, 15 years ago gallbladders were removed by using open surgery. Patients stayed in the hospital for 7 to 10 days and recovered at home for 6 weeks. Now, gallbladders are removed laparoscopically, the patient may stay in the hospital overnight, and then recover for a week or two at home. For anti-reflux surgery, make sure your surgeon is comfortable performing laparoscopic surgery and has performed at least 20 laparoscopic anti-reflux surgeries, because there is a learning curve and practice is important.

Medicine is a business, and surgeons are paid to operate—this could create a conflict of interest. Your surgeon should be methodical in the approach to surgery, ensuring that your evaluation prior to surgery is complete. As previously discussed, a full evaluation generally includes endoscopy, motility studies, and pH studies. These tests help to confirm the diagnosis of GERD, assess any damage to the esophagus, and improve surgical results. Anti-reflux surgery is elective surgery, and you should be leery if a surgeon tries to rush you into making a decision or cuts any corners during presurgery evaluation. Ask your surgeon about his or her experience and how patients have done and what complications they have had.

*Anti-reflux surgery is elective surgery, and you should be leery if a surgeon tries to rush you into making a decision or cuts any corners during presurgery evaluation.*

## 95. What are the endoscopic therapies for GERD?

Technology is always improving, and doctors are always looking for better and different techniques to solve problems. Over the last 8 years, several nonsurgical procedures have been developed to strengthen the lower esophageal sphincter and treat reflux. All of these techniques involve endoscopy with modification of the tools usually used. One method to tighten the LES is injection of material into the region of the LES to bulk it up; this therapy is called Enteryx. Another technique uses radiofrequency ablation that damages or "cooks" the LES, causing scarring and contraction of the area, which tightens it; this procedure is called Stretta. Several techniques similar to a Nissen fundoplication wrap the stomach around the bottom of the esophagus and stitch it in place using the endoscope. These techniques are all different but have a similar result and are called the NDO Plicator, Bard EndoCinch, and the Wilson-Cook Endoscopic Suturing Device. All of these endoscopic therapies are FDA approved and are in use. They are discussed separately in the following questions.

## 96. What is a Stretta procedure?

Generally, a weak or lax lower esophageal sphincter causes reflux, although some reflux is related to inappropriate relaxation of the LES. Historically, anti-reflux surgical procedures wrap part of the stomach around the LES to tighten or reinforce this region. As mentioned earlier, several techniques have been developed to accomplish this nonoperatively with an endoscope to avoid the risks and discomfort of surgery.

When tissue is damaged, it scars and shortens or contracts and becomes stiffer. When the body repairs a wound, it uses a material it produces called collagen. Collagen in your body provides strength and elasticity to tissues. As you age, for example, collagen breaks down and leads to wrinkles; also, plastic surgeons use collagen injections to treat wrinkles.

A Stretta procedure uses this concept of scarring and collagen production to reinforce the lower esophageal sphincter (see Figure 15). First, the patient is heavily sedated or given general anesthesia and undergoes a regular endoscopy test. Then, the endoscope is

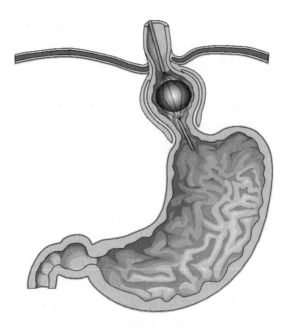

**Figure 15    Stretta.**

removed and a probe is placed in the esophagus at the level of the LES. This tool has several needles sticking out to pierce the wall of the esophagus. When in place, radiofrequency energy (like that used in a microwave oven) is passed down the probe and out the needles into the esophageal wall. This causes the local temperature of the tissues to increase, virtually to the point of "cooking" or damaging the area. The probe is repositioned several times, and the procedure of radiofrequency ablation is repeated until the whole LES is treated. Overall, this takes 30 to 60 minutes. The result is, hopefully, uniform damage to the LES, which heals over time with scarring and increased collagen production, which thereby tightens the LES.

Several studies have examined patients who have had Stretta procedures. Most patients were able to stop or reduce their use of proton pump inhibitor medication.

Most patients would recommend this procedure to a friend or undergo the procedure again. In a small study of patients, pH studies demonstrated an improvement in the amount and duration of acid in the esophagus. Complications of the procedure include chest pain requiring narcotics, damage to the lining of the esophagus, and difficulty swallowing. In the first 6 months of use, four perforations of the esophagus (a hole through the esophageal wall) and two deaths from aspiration pneumonia occurred. The overall serious complication rate is about 1 in 400.

Generally, radiofrequency ablation or Stretta is for patients who have failed to improve with medication and who do not want or cannot have a surgical repair of the LES. Stretta is not suitable for those patients with large hiatal hernias. It is a fairly new procedure and the long-term risks and benefits and ability to stay off medication really are unknown. Stretta is FDA approved and is currently available.

## 97. What is Enteryx?

Enteryx is a material that could be injected into the area of the LES at the time of endoscopy. It is a liquid polymer that stays in place where it is injected and solidifies into a spongy material. This material can bulk up the LES and become a barrier to reflux. Small studies suggested that Enteryx was effective for GERD. Side effects included chest pain, difficulty swallowing, bloating, nausea, garlic odor, and fever.

Enteryx was previously FDA approved, but because of complications (11 esophageal perforations and one death reported) it was removed from the market on October 14, 2005. Enteryx is no longer approved for use in the Unites States.

## 98. What is an EndoCinch or endoscopic plication?

A Nissen fundoplication is, as mentioned earlier, surgical reinforcement of the lower esophageal sphincter accomplished by wrapping the top of the stomach around the bottom of the esophagus and stitching it into place. Several companies have manufactured endoscopic devices that can sew or staple and effectively provide a similar effect as a Nissen procedure. Currently, three endoscopic stitching or sewing devices are approved by the FDA and are on the market. Each device is different and requires a different technique to deliver a suture or stitch, but the results are roughly the same.

The Bard EndoCinch has been on the market since 2000 and is the most studied and tested of the devices mentioned here (see Figure 16). A complicated technique of placing several stitches in the region of the esophagogastric junction is required. Studies on patient outcome are limited. In a 2-year study of 85 patients who had the procedure, more than half of the patients reported improved GERD symptoms and more than 40% did not require PPI medication at 2 years.

Another sewing device is the NDO Surgical Plicator. The plicator is another nonsurgical, endoscopy-assisted technique to tighten the LES. This device is FDA approved and is currently available. Studies of patient outcome at 1 year suggest similar results as those obtained with the Bard EndoCinch in terms of acid control and need for medication.

The third device is the Wilson-Cook Endoscopic Suturing Device. It is used in an endoscopy-assisted and nonsurgical procedure to tighten the LES. This

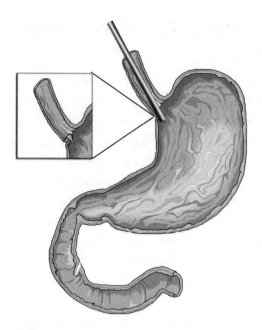

**Figure 16    Endocinch.**

device is FDA approved and is commercially available; however, there is very little human data regarding outcome.

It is interesting to note that the FDA regulates all prescribed drugs and surgical devices in the United States. For a new drug to become FDA approved, hundreds of millions of dollars are spent by a drug company. The drug is tested for years for safety, efficacy (meaning it works for the illness it was made for), and appropriate dosing. Then, the drug is approved and followed to see whether any new side effects or bad reactions are reported when it is marketed to the public and thousands or millions of people take it. At any point in the process, the FDA can step in and stop or remove a drug from the market. Several drugs underwent years of testing only to be removed from sales in the United

States. Some of the most notable are thalidomide, which caused birth defects; dexfenfluramine (Redux) for weight loss, which may have caused heart problems; and rofecoxib (Vioxx), an arthritis drug which may increase risk of heart attacks.

This, however, does not apply to surgical devices, which are approved by the FDA after little testing. Really, only when the device is out on the market and being used are side effects and complications found. This is the case for endoscopic or noninvasive anti-reflux procedures. These technologies are FDA approved only after they are documented to work and are shown to be safe for a small number of test subjects. The demonstration of safety and long-term benefit comes after they are out and used on thousands of people. It was this postmarketing safety information that led the FDA to remove Enteryx from the market.

## 99. Who performs noninvasive, endoscopic anti-reflux procedures?

These procedures are widely available and are commercially available by all doctors. Any gastroenterologist or surgeon who wants to do something different or offer a procedure that others do not offer may perform these procedures. If you are to undergo a noninvasive anti-reflux procedure, make sure it is done by a doctor who has performed it many times and has experience. Such doctors generally can be found in large hospitals or teaching hospitals. They may have participated in testing of the device prior to FDA approval and may have the greatest experience with the new device.

The problem is there is potential for abuse of the technology by doctors. For example, the Enteryx injection procedure does not require any special machines or instruments and really can be done by anyone who can perform an endoscopy. The ability to inject medication with an endoscope is easy, and physicians do it commonly. Enteryx is simply a different material to be injected into a specific place. This technique was widely used by doctors at smaller and community hospitals without adequate experience or backup. Ultimately, it led to severe complications and even death in some patients, so the company that produced it and the FDA removed the material from the market.

## 100. What are the long-term risks/benefits of endoscopic anti-reflux procedures?

The short answer is we really do not know the long-term risks of endoscopic anti-reflux procedures because they have only been on the market for a few years. Likewise, we do not know their long-term durability to control GERD symptoms and provide heartburn relief without medications. These are promising technologies that make sense from a medical standpoint, but they have not yet stood the test of time. Because these technologies are still fairly new, think carefully before you have your esophagus plicated or ablated by radiofrequency. GERD, for the most part, is a benign but inconvenient condition. These procedures have risks that can be life threatening, and the long-term outcome is unknown. To date, endoscopic anti-reflux procedures are not the **standard of care**. (Standard of care is what the average doctor would do or what is expected of most doctors.) The current standard of care for someone who has long-term

*These are promising technologies that make sense from a medical standpoint, but they have not yet stood the test of time.*

GERD is medication, and if that fails, open or laparoscopic surgery would be the next option.

Richard's comment:

*I have had symptoms of acid reflux for more than 10 years. Most of my acid reflux incidents occur during the evening while I sleep. Although the symptoms have increased over the years, so has my age and the reasons that cause acid reflux (late meals, added weight, late-night snacks, lack of exercise, etc.). When I adhere to a schedule that includes taking my medication regularly, eating properly, eating smaller meals at the appropriate times, and staying away from processed foods, chocolate, and fatty snacks, I would never know I have acid reflux. Therefore, for me a lifestyle change is what I need to control my acid reflux, not surgery.*

# PART ELEVEN

# *Conclusion and Summary Thoughts*

### *Bonus Question: What would I do if I had chronic GERD?*

DLB answers: This is a good question because I have had GERD almost daily for the last 20 years. I take my medication every day, and it controls my symptoms. And if I miss a dose, I know it. Lifestyle modification truly helps, and the greatest benefit is avoiding food for 2 hours prior to bed. Given the lack of long-term documented benefit of endoscopic anti-reflux procedures, I would not have one and do not recommend these procedures to my patients. As for anti-reflux surgery, well, surgery has risks and complications. The long-term benefit of a Nissen procedure performed either openly or laparoscopically is roughly equal to that of medication.

And frequently, those who have had the surgery need to go back to their medication. The disadvantage to this approach is the need to take regular medicine and its associated cost. So, my usual recommendation to my patients and what I do for myself is stick to the medication because it is safe for long-term use and effective in controlling GERD symptoms.

# *Appendix*

**About GERD**
Sponsored by the International Foundation for Functional Gastrointestinal
    Disorders, Inc.
Web site: www.aboutgerd.org

**EMedicineHealth.com**
Web site: www.emedicinehealth.com/script/main/art.asp?articlekey=60061

**Gastroesophageal Reflux Disease**
Sponsored by Wikipedia, the Free Encyclopedia
Web site: http://en.wikipedia.org/wiki/GERD (case sensitive)

**GERD Information Resource Center**
Sponsored by AstraZeneca
Web site: www.gerd.com

**MayoClinic.com**
Web site: www.mayoclinic.com/health/heartburn-gerd/DS00095

**MedicineNet.com**
Web site: www.medicinenet.com/gastroesophageal_reflux_disease_gerd/
    article.htm

**National Digestive Diseases Information Clearinghouse (NDDIC)**
Sponsored by National Institutes of Health
Web site: http://digestive.niddk.nih.gov/ddiseases/pubs/gerd

Appendix

# *Glossary*

**Adenocarcinoma:** Two types of cancer occur in the esophagus. Adenocarcinoma is a certain type of cancer characterized by the presence of glands when examined under the microscope. This is the kind of cancer associated with Barrett's esophagus.

**Alka Seltzer:** A brand of antacid medication that effervesces. An antacid that contains aspirin.

**Anemia:** A low blood count from either blood loss or inadequate blood production.

**Antacid:** A medication available over the counter, effective for active symptoms of reflux. Antacids work by neutralizing acid on contact. Many types of antacid medications are available without a doctor's prescription.

**Aspiration:** The process of food or liquid entering the airway or lungs. Aspiration can occur on swallowing and commonly happens in patients who have had prior strokes and who cannot swallow normally. Aspiration can also occur accompanying GERD. The refluxed material comes up through the esophagus to the mouth and then may be inhaled, damaging the airways (trachea or larynx) or lungs. Aspiration can result in severe pneumonias.

**Balloon dilator:** A balloon on the end of a long thin tube that goes down the endoscope.

**Barium study or swallow:** An X-ray test in which barium, a liquid that can be seen on X rays, is swallowed, and X-ray pictures are taken to see whether there are any abnormalities of the esophagus, stomach, or duodenum. A barium study is a very helpful test for patients with chronic GERD and difficulty swallowing. The barium study can help differentiate a benign stricture from a cancer.

**Barrett's esophagus:** An inflammatory condition of the esophagus caused by chronic gastroesophageal reflux disease. Barrett's esophagus is a more acid-resistant lining of the esophagus that can predispose a person to the development of esophageal cancer.

**Bernstein test:** Acid (like stomach acid) is infused into the esophagus during a motility test. This allows for pressure measurement in the esophagus to see if muscle spasms occur and the patient can subjectively tell the tester whether he or she is having chest pain during the acid challenge.

**Biopsy:** A small tissue sample that can be studied under the microscope.

**Body mass index (BMI):** A standardized measure of weight for height. It is calculated by dividing weight in kilograms by height in meters squared.

**Diaphragm:** The main muscle that controls breathing. The diaphragm is a muscle that separates the chest from the abdomen. The esophagus passes through a hole in the diaphragm called a hiatus to reach the stomach in the abdomen.

**Dilator:** A tool usually used at the time of endoscopy to stretch out esophageal rings or strictures to improve swallowing. *See* Balloon dilator.

**DNA:** Deoxyribonucleic acid. The genetic code within all living cells that regulates cell reproduction and differentiation (what kind of cell a cell becomes).

**Duodenum:** The first part of the small intestine starting at the end of the stomach.

**Dysphagia:** Difficulty swallowing; the sensation during swallowing of food getting stuck somewhere in the neck or chest.

**Dysplasia:** Tissue changes seen under a microscope that show the degeneration toward cancer. Dysplasia is not cancer but a preliminary stage that can become cancer. In Barrett's esophagus, the presence of dysplasia means the patient has an increased risk of developing cancer. Dysplasia can be mild (called low-grade dysplasia) or severe (known as high-grade dysplasia), and management of these conditions is different.

**Endoscope:** An instrument used to examine the esophagus, stomach, and small intestine. A long, thin camera with a light source that can be steered once inserted and can enable the physician to take pictures and perform biopsies.

**Endoscopy center:** A place where endoscopies are performed, either at a hospital or not associated with a hospital. A center not at a hospital is called an ambulatory or outpatient endoscopy center.

**Enteric coating:** A coating applied to capsules that allows the capsule to disintegrate in the small intestine instead of the stomach.

**Esophageal dilation:** The technique of stretching the esophagus, it is used to treat difficulty swallowing caused by structures or rings.

**Esophagitis:** Inflammation of the lining of the esophagus that is present in about half of those with chronic reflux symptoms. Esophagitis is diagnosed either by performing a barium study or by endoscopy. Symptoms of esophagitis are heartburn and occasional difficulty swallowing, and it is treated with proton pump inhibitors or H2 blockers.

**Esophagus:** A long muscular tube that runs from the throat down to the stomach that allows passage of food from the mouth to the stomach. The esophagus passes through the chest behind the heart and through the diaphragm to join the stomach.

**Event recorder:** A small electrical recording device that is generally worn on a patient's belt and that is connected to a measuring instrument such as a pH probe. The event recorder records the acid measurements in the esophagus and has a button the patient can press to note when he or she experiences GERD symptoms. When the study is complete, the event recorder is connected to a computer and the acid measurements and patient symptoms are analyzed.

**Fizzy:** A material that produces gas and helps to distend your stomach so it can be more carefully examined.

**Forceps:** A long, thin tool that is passed down the endoscope to take biopsies.

**Gastric:** Of or relating to the stomach.

**Gastroenterologist:** A doctor who specializes in diseases and disorders of the gastrointestinal tract. This includes diseases of the esophagus, stomach, intestine, colon, liver, and pancreas. A doctor who treats GERD and performs endoscopy.

**Gastroesophageal junction (GEJ):** The junction of the stomach and esophagus where the lining or mucosa changes. The region of the lower esophageal sphincter.

**GERD:** Gastroesophageal reflux disease. A disease made up of symptoms of heartburn, reflux, and/or regurgitation.

**Goblet cells:** A certain kind of cell present in the gut but not normally found in the esophagus. Its presence is required for the pathologist to make the diagnosis of specialized intestinal metaplasia or Barrett's esophagus.

**H2 blocker:** A drug that generally does not require a prescription and is available over the counter. These drugs decrease acid production by the stomach. H2 blockers are effective for esophagitis, GERD, and peptic ulcer disease. They are best used to prevent GERD symptoms and are safe for long-term use. Examples are ranitidine (Zantac), famotidine (Pepcid), nizatidine (Axid), and cimetidine (Tagamet).

**Heartburn:** The sensation of burning discomfort or warmth traveling up from the stomach into the chest. A symptom of GERD.

***Helicobacter pylori (H. pylori)*:** A bacterium that lives in the stomach and can cause stomach ulcers. It is diagnosed usually by biopsy of the stomach and treated with 10 to 14 days of antibiotics and antacid medication. The role of *H. pylori* in GERD is unclear.

**Hiatal hernia or hiatus hernia**: The chest and abdomen are separated by a muscle for breathing called the diaphragm. The gastroesophageal junction (GEJ) is level with the diaphragm, meaning the esophagus is in the chest above the diaphragm and the stomach is below it in the abdomen. To pass into the chest the esophagus travels through a hole in the diaphragm. Sometimes this hole becomes too large and the top of the stomach can herniate, or pass, into the chest. This condition is called a hiatal hernia. A hiatal hernia causes a weakening in the lower esophageal sphincter and is associated with reflux. There are two types of hiatal hernias—sliding and paraesophageal.

**Hiatus**: A naturally occurring hole in a bodily structure or a passageway through a bodily structure. For example, the hiatus of the diaphragm is where the esophagus passes from the chest into the abdomen.

**High-grade dysplasia (HGD)**: Microscopic changes in Barrett's esophagus that may become cancerous. High-grade dysplasia is not frankly cancerous. However, cancer can exist in the setting of HGD. High-grade dysplasia needs to be confirmed by two different pathologists who examine the tissue. If HGD is found, then surgery with removal of the esophagus may be recommended.

**Histamine**: A substance normally produced by the body that can stimulate stomach acid production. A substance also responsible for allergic reactions.

**Histamine-2 receptor antagonist**: *See* H2 blocker.

**Informed consent**: The process of explaining the reason for performing a procedure and the risks associated with it. The doctor usually goes over this information before doing a procedure. The patient must then read and sign a permission form for the procedure.

**Larynx**: A structure in the throat; the beginning of the airway located at the top of the trachea. The larynx is also known as the voice box. The larynx can be affected in GERD with resulting voice changes, irritation, and on rare occasions, cancer.

**Los Angeles Esophagitis Grading Scale**: A grading scale used at the time of endoscopy to describe the severity of damage to or inflammation of the esophagus. There are four grades, A through D. Grade A is mild inflammation with patchy redness, and grade D is severe inflammation with ulcers.

**Low-grade dysplasia (LGD)**: Microscopic changes in Barrett's esophagus that may become cancerous. Low-grade dysplasia is not cancer. The presence of LGD increases the need for periodic or surveillance endoscopy to one every year.

**Lower esophageal ring (LER)**: A narrowing at the bottom of the esophagus that can cause difficulty in swallowing. A lower esophageal ring is treated at the time of endoscopy by dilating it to improve swallowing.

**Lower esophageal sphincter (LES):** A circular muscle at the bottom of the esophagus above the stomach. This muscle opens when food enters the esophagus, allowing the food passage into the stomach, and contracts, or closes, in between swallows. This muscle, or sphincter, may be too loose or may open at inappropriate times, allowing material to reflux from the stomach up into the esophagus.

**Malaise:** A vague sense of being ill.

**Maloney dilator:** A tool used at the time of endoscopy to dilate or stretch out narrowing or strictures in the esophagus to improve swallowing.

**Manometry study:** *See* Motility study.

**Motility study:** A test used to evaluate GERD. A small tube is placed in the esophagus, and pressures are measured during swallowing to ensure that muscle contractions in the esophagus are appropriate and effective. This test is usually performed at a hospital or endoscopy center.

**Mucosa:** The lining of the gut. Each gut organ has a special mucosa that can be identified under the microscope. The mucosa is like the "skin" lining the gut.

**Nissen fundoplication:** Wrapping the top of the stomach all the way around the bottom of the esophagus to tighten the LES.

**Nonsteroidal anti-inflammatory drugs (NSAIDs):** A class of medication generally used to treat pain. All NSAIDs can cause irritation or ulcers of the gastrointestinal tract. Examples are aspirin, ibuprofen (Motrin, Advil), and naproxen (Aleve).

**Obese:** Roughly 30 pounds overweight.

**Over-the-counter medication:** A medication that does not require a doctor's prescription and is available at the pharmacy.

**Paraesophageal hernia:** A rare type of hiatal hernia that can occur in the elderly. A paraesophageal hernia is a sliding hiatal hernia in which part of the stomach herniates into the chest next to the esophagus. Because of its location in the chest this part of the stomach is vulnerable to losing its blood supply and usually requires surgery to fix.

**Parietal cell:** A cell within the stomach that produces acid and is responsible for normal absorption of vitamin $B_{12}$.

**Pathologist:** A doctor who specializes in the study of tissues or cells. A doctor who performs autopsies.

**pH:** A grading scale that determines the amount of acid or base a solid or liquid contains.

**pH study or test:** A test used to diagnose GERD. A small tube is placed in the esophagus and generally is left in place for 24 hours. This tube measures the amount and duration of acid in the esophagus. It is connected to a small event monitor that records the amount of acid and that has a button that allows the patient to note when he or she is having reflux symptoms. The tube is usually placed at a doctor's office or endoscopy center and is worn home and then returned the next day.

**Pharynx:** A structure in the throat. The beginning of the digestive system located at the top of the esophagus.

**Pill ulcer:** Ulcer caused by taking an aspirin or ibuprofen at bedtime without drinking enough water. The pill then sits in the esophagus all night, burning a hole in the lining.

**PPI:** *See* Proton pump inhibitor.

**Proton pump inhibitor:** A drug that blocks acid production by the stomach; believed to be stronger and more effective than H2 blockers are. The most effective medication available to treat acid damage to the esophagus and GERD. Generally recommended for those with severe GERD, esophageal strictures, or Barrett's esophagus. An over-the-counter example is Prilosec. Prescription examples are omeprazole, esomeprazole (Nexium), pantoprazole (Protonix), and lansoprazole (Prevacid).

**Reflux:** The movement of food, fluid, or acid up from the stomach into the esophagus.

**Regurgitation:** The symptom of "burping" up material or the movement of material up from the stomach to the esophagus and then into the mouth. Regurgitation can cause a bitter taste in the mouth, and chronic symptoms can cause damage to the teeth or bad breath.

**Sliding hiatal hernia:** The most common type of hiatal hernia in which part of the stomach slides from the abdomen into the chest. *See also* Hiatal hernia.

**Sorbitol:** A sweetener used in foods, candies, and medications. A sugar that can cause diarrhea.

**Specialized intestinal metaplasia:** An abnormal lining of the esophagus that can be seen under the microscope by a pathologist. Specialized intestinal metaplasia is the finding used to diagnose Barrett's esophagus.

**Squamous cell carcinoma:** A type of cancer that can occur in many areas. The commonly seen cancer in the head and neck or esophagus associated with smoking. Under the microscope, there are no glands. Squamous cell carcinoma can occur in the esophagus, but adenocarcinoma is associated with Barrett's esophagus.

**Standard of care:** What the average doctor would do or what is expected of most doctors.

**Steakhouse syndrome:** Symptoms of relatively rare difficulty swallowing with the sensation of food getting stuck. Classically, steakhouse syndrome occurs when a person has had a few alcoholic drinks, is eating meat, and eats too quickly or does not chew the food carefully. Then the meat gets stuck above a lower esophageal ring upon swallowing.

**Stricture:** A narrowing of the esophagus. Generally causes difficulty swallowing.

**Trachea:** A structure within the chest. The main airway leading from the throat to the lungs.

**Transfat:** A fat usually present in fast food. Transfat should be consumed in small amounts as it is felt to be primarily responsible for increasing the risk of heart disease and certain cancers.

**Ulcer:** An area of damage or a break in the lining of the gut. An ulcer can occur anywhere in the gastrointestinal tract. Classically, ulcers occur in the stomach or duodenum.

**Upper esophageal sphincter (UES):** A circular muscle at the top of the esophagus that is usually closed and relaxes on swallowing, allowing passage of material from the mouth into the esophagus. The UES also protects from reflux traveling up from the esophagus into the mouth or airways.

**Upper GI series:** A barium examination of the esophagus, stomach, and duodenum. *See* Barium study.

**Urease breath test:** Testing breath after mildly radioactive urea is consumed.

# *Index*

esophageal motility testing, 94
esophageal perforations, 78–79, 107–108
esophageal rings, 74–75
esophageal strictures, 76
  seeing during endoscopy, 112
esophageal ulcers, 118–119
  defined, 174
esophagitis, 6, 72–74, 100, 170
  risks after surgery, 152
esophagus, 171
  anatomy of, 5, 19
  biopsies of. *See* biopsy
  cancer of. *See* cancer (esophageal)
  damage to. *See* complications of
    GERD
  medications that affect, 3, 20, 44–54
  narrowing of. *See* LER (lower
    esophageal ring)
  nicotine effects, 43
estrogen, 15–16, 49
evaluation by doctor, 98–102
  before surgery, 147–148
event recorder, 115–116, 171
exercise, 54–56
  reducing cancer risk, 87

**F**

family history. *See* genetic predisposition
famotidine (Pepcid), 132. *See also* H2 blockers
fast food, 11, 13, 59–61
fat, dietary, 11, 55, 56, 58, 62. *See also* diet
    and nutrition
  fast food, 60
FDA (Food & Drug Administration), 159
felodipine (Plendil), 47
fentanyl. *See* narcotics
fillers in medications, 129
fizzies, 104, 171
Fluxid (famotidine), 132. *See also* H2 blockers
foods. *See* diet and nutrition
forceps, defined, 171
Fosamax (alendronate sodium), 49, 76. *See
    also* osteoporosis, drugs for
fruits and vegetables, eating, 58

**G**

garlic, 57. *See also* diet and nutrition
gastric, defined, 171
gastroenterologists, 99, 105, 171
gastroesophageal junction (GEJ), 112, 171

gastroesophageal reflux disease. *See* entries
    at GERD
GEJ (gastroesophageal junction), 112, 171
genetic predisposition, 10
  as reason for endoscopy, 113
geography, likelihood of GERD and, 7–8
GERD, defined, 2–3, 171
GERD, prevalence of, 6–8
GERD complications. *See* complications of
    GERD
GERD symptoms. *See* symptoms of
    GERD; treatment of GERD
goblet cells, 80, 171
gravity, role of, 19, 34, 65

**H**

*H. pylori* (*Helicobacter pylori*), 110, 120–124,
    171
H2 blockers, 67, 72, 74, 131–134
  antacids vs., 127
  for children, 14
  defined, 171, 172
  how to take, 139–141
  PPIs vs., 132–134
  side effects of, 137–139
  taking for life, 146
  treating *H. pylori*, 124
  trying out, 101
  when not working, 141–142
  when to take, 140
halitosis (symptom), 32
health insurance, medication and, 67–68
heart attacks, 26, 93
heartburn, 3, 4, 17
  defined, 171
  differentiating from heart problems,
    26–27
  medications that cause, 47
  from stress, 42
*Helicobacter pylori* (*H. pylori*), 110, 120–124,
    120–124, 171
hereditary predisposition, 10
  as reason for endoscopy, 113
HGD (high-grade dysplasia), defined, 172
hiatal hernia, 9–10, 19, 38–40
  aging and, 63
  defined, 38–39, 171
  symptoms and complications, 39–40
hiatus, 19, 172
high-blood-pressure medications, 21, 44, 48
high-grade dysplasia (HGD), 172
high-pressure zone, 9

Index

rofecoxib (Vioxx), 161
Rolaids. *See* antacids

## S

saliva, 18
saliva production, 33
    aging and, 18, 63
    cigarette smoke and, 43–44
salt consumption, 60
sedatives, 48, 49
    for endoscopy, 106, 107
seriousness of GERD, 16, 35–36, 70
side effects of medications, 137–139. *See also*
    *specific medication by name or type*
silent symptoms (silent reflux), 30–32
Sinemet (levodopa), 47
Sinequan (doxepin), 47
sippy diet, 58
skin rashes, 30
sleep habits, 20–21, 65. *See also* nighttime
    symptoms
    aspiration, 89
    preventing aspiration, 89
sliding hiatal hernia, 39, 174. *See also* hiatal
    hernia
smoking, 22, 43–44, 90, 95
    reducing cancer risk, 86–87
smooth muscle, 45, 46
sodas. *See* carbonated beverages
sodium, in antacids, 128
sorbitol, 129–130, 174
soy products, eating, 59
specialized intestinal metaplasia, 80, 174
spicy foods, 56, 57. *See also* diet and nutrition
squamous cell carcinoma, 81, 174
standard of care, 162–163, 174
steakhouse syndrome, 74–75, 174
stomach. *See also* LES (lower esophageal
    sphincter)
    anatomy of, 5, 19
    medications that affect, 50–51
    mucosa, 50, 111–112, 173
    role of, 38
stopping medication, 143–144
stress, 42
Stretta procedure, 156–158
    long-term risks and benefits, 162
    who performs, 161
stricture, 18, 174
strictures, esophageal, 76
    seeing during endoscopy, 112

sugars in antacids, 129
Sumycin (tetracycline). *See* antibiotics
super-sizing. *See* fast food
surgery for GERD, 147–149, 147–155
    FDA regulation, 160
    finding a surgeon, 154–155
    long-term benefits, 150–152
    medications vs., 152–153, 165–166
swallowing problems, 17–18, 100–101
    steakhouse syndrome, 74–75, 174
    studying. *See* motility testing (manometry studies)
sweets, eating, 59
symptoms of esophageal cancer, 85–86
symptoms of esophagitis, 71
symptoms of GERD, 17–18, 21–23. *See also*
    treatment of GERD
    after surgery, 151
    alarm signs, 35–36, 85–86, 100–101, 138
    chest pain, diagnosing, 26–30
    in children, 14
    daytime vs. nighttime GERD, 33–35.
      *See also* bedtime symptoms
    drugs for. *See* medications
    laryngeal cancer, 35, 90, 95
    medical evaluation, getting, 98–102, 147–148
    mouth symptoms, 31–32
    no symptoms (silent), 30–32
    stopping medication, 143–144
    from stress, 42–43
    voice-related, 29
    when to get endoscopy, 112–113
symptoms of hiatal hernia, 39–40

## T

Tagamet (cimetidine), 132. *See also* H2
    blockers
teeth-related symptoms, 31, 32
testing for GERD, 104–116. *See also* diagnosing GERD
    barium studies, 104, 113, 169
    biopsy. *See* biopsy
    endoscopy. *See* endoscopy
    manometry studies (motility testing), 94, 113–115, 148, 173
    pH studies, 91, 93, 94, 115–116, 148, 173
testing for *H. pylori*, 122–123
tetracycline (Sumycin). *See* antibiotics
thalidomide, 161

theophylline, 47, 48
Tiazac (diltiazem), 47
tobacco (smoking), 22, 43–44, 90, 95
    reducing cancer risk, 86–87
Tofranil (imipramine), 47, 49
tofu, 59
tomato-based foods, 57. *See also* diet and
    nutrition
tooth-related symptoms, 31, 32
Toprol (metoprolol), 47
Toupet procedure, 150
trachea, 28, 174
trachea, liquids entering. *See* aspiration
trans fat, 60, 174
treatment for *H. pylori*, 123–124
treatment of GERD, 21–23
    endoscopic therapies, 155–163
    medications, when to take, 66–68
    surgery, 147–155
tricyclic antidepressants. *See* depression
    medications
Tums (calcium carbonate), 67, 127. *See also*
    antacids

**U**

UES (upper esophageal sphincter), 114, 175
ulcers, 118–119
    defined, 174
uneasiness (symptom), 17
Uniphyl (theophylline), 47
upper endoscopy. *See* endoscopy
upper esophageal sphincter (UES), 114,
    175
upper GI series. *See* barium studies
urease breath test, 122–123, 175

**V**

Valium (diazepam), 47
vegetables and fruits, eating, 58
verapamil (Calan), 48. *See also* blood pres-
    sure drugs
Vioxx (rofecoxib), 161
visiting a doctor, 98–102
    before surgery, 147–148
vitamin B$_{12}$ deficiency, 146
vitamin C supplements, 77
voice-related symptoms, 29, 31, 35, 90

**W**

warning signs. *See* alarm signs
water brash, 33
water, taking with medications, 52–53
wedge pillows, 21, 34, 65
    preventing aspiration, 89
weight gain and obesity. *See* body weight
    and obesity
Wilson-Cook Endoscopic Suturing Device,
    158–159
windpipe (trachea), 28, 174
women, GERD in, 15–16

**Y**

yogurt, eating, 59

**Z**

Zantac (ranitidine), 132. *See also* H2 block-
    ers
Zegerid (omeprazole), 101, 135. *See also*
    PPIs
Zithromax, 77. *See also* antibiotics